Praise for
NATURALLY THIN

"I really want to thank you for your book and I have to tell you your book saved me. I no longer hyperventilate when going out to eat, or freak out about not being able to work out every day . . . I know I did the work and I am proud of myself for what I've accomplished, but, Bethenny, your book was exactly what I needed to really, finally, totally, resolve my issues with food." —*Angelique*

"I just wanted to thank you for changing my life . . . probably a bit extreme but I truly don't think about food the same way after reading your book. Your words made so much sense to me that I started living by them immediately. That was three months ago and I very easily dropped 15 pounds." —*Kim*

"At 24 I'm pretty sure that I've tried 24 different diets. *Naturally Thin* has taught me tools that are life-changing. 'You can have it all, just not all at once' and 'Check yourself before you wreck yourself' are two of the most important concepts for me. When my 'food noise' is telling me to have a greasy burrito and to just start over tomorrow—I can literally hear Bethenny saying the titles of the chapters in my head. And then I'm able to move on. Despite the weight loss, I am most proud of how I feel in control. Oh yeah, and I've lost 30 pounds!"
—*Krystal*, New York, New York

"I bought your book on Friday, finished reading it on Saturday morning, and by Wednesday I had already lost 2 pounds! The way that I thought about food needed to be altered and you helped me do that with your ten rules and two key (genius) concepts. Your book is fun, smart, straightforward, and REAL, just like you."
—*Dana*, Milpitas, California

"I now feel like I may actually have a shot at taking back my life. It is MINE after all, and you have already made it seem like something I can do. Thank you for not setting another unattainable goal for real people." —*Erin*, New York, New York

"The best part is that my boyfriend is totally on board. I think he's relieved that he doesn't have to deal with a girl who's dieting, and that makes HIS life easier . . . and so from time to time (in a terrifically supportive way) he'll mention one of the 10 rules that applies to the moment I'm dealing with. This is great—relatable and easy." —*Darby*

"I just purchased your book and read it from cover to cover in two days. Now I am not an avid or fast reader so this speaks volumes. I felt touched, moved, and inspired with every word on every page. There were even sections that brought tears to my eyes. It was like you were in my own head full knowing and speaking directly to my own personal struggles with the obsessing then binging vicious cycle."

—*Therese*

"I'm a 21-year-old student that has been struggling with eating issues for 2 years. I picked up your *Naturally Thin* book at the store the other day and I am halfway through. I am amazed by how much I relate to EVERYTHING you say . . . I wanted to let you know your book is amazing and is helping me find a healthy relationship with food! I am currently in therapy for my obsession, but I feel as if your book is helping me so much more. I'm sure many others feel this way. I look up to you so much!"

—*Anonymous*

"Thank you so much, Bethenny, for your book. It has really changed my life and I can already feel with certainty that these changes will last forever. I have thrown all my other diet books out the door. I have been gaining and losing the same 30 pounds all my adult life (mostly gaining). I bought your book the week it came out, and now I am 25 pounds thinner, binge free, guilt free, food obsession gone, eating healthy, and I'm on top of the world." —*Debbie*, Mt. Laurel, New Jersey

"Since reading your book, I have been waking up every day inspired and encouraged. You've made it so easy to understand and grasp the tools and tips offered in your book, and I'm learning to use them on a daily basis. I also love your easy recipes that you've included in your book, which I find to be an added bonus. Your wonderful personality shines throughout *Naturally Thin* and I thank you, thank you from the bottom of my heart! Bethenny, you've changed my life."

—*Gina*, Tulsa, Oklahoma

"I did not pick up your book for diet reasons but rather medical ones. I figured I'd let you know that you aren't only addressing the 'struggling to be thin' community, but also those with medical issues pertaining to the stomach, *and* my battle with food; something I was losing. I picked up your book for the natural recipes, but what I got instead was a lot more." —*Laura*, New York, New York

"I have my master's in psychotherapy and have studied for years the relationship between what we eat and how we feel. I am opening a clinic here in Phoenix, with a naturopathic physician, nutritionist, acupuncturist, TCM, etc., under one roof, designed to get people healthy naturally. Bethenny has spoken to me through the book in a funny but intellectual way. Too often, nutritionists and/or chefs write these books and they're missing something: personality and ease. If people are intimidated, or uninterested to read something, what good is the information? I have a feeling Bethenny's book will fill this gap for years to come."

—*Molly*, Phoenix, Arizona

"Your book has changed my life forever. I am 38 and am finally free from food prison. I have lost weight without even trying. Where have you been all my life?"

—*Suzanne*, Marietta, Georgia

Also by Bethenny Frankel

NATURALLY THIN

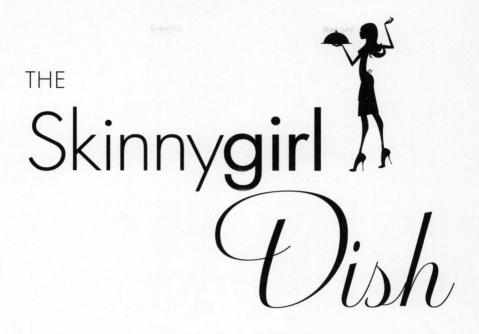

THE

Skinnygirl

Dish

Easy Recipes for Your
Naturally Thin Life

BETHENNY FRANKEL

with Eve Adamson

A Fireside Book
Published by Simon & Schuster
NEW YORK   LONDON   TORONTO   SYDNEY

Fireside
A Division of Simon & Schuster, Inc.
1230 Avenue of the Americas
New York, NY 10020

First Fireside trade paperback edition January 2010

FIRESIDE and colophon are registered trademarks of Simon & Schuster, Inc.

For information about special discounts for bulk purchases,
please contact Simon & Schuster Special Sales at
1-866-506-1949 or business@simonandschuster.com.

The Simon & Schuster Speakers Bureau can bring authors to your live event.
For more information or to book an event, contact the Simon & Schuster Speakers
Bureau at 1-866-248-3049 or visit our website at www.simonspeakers.com.

Designed by Joy O'Meara
Illustration from iStockphoto.com

Manufactured in the United States of America

10   9   8   7   6   5   4   3   2   1

Library of Congress Cataloging-in-Publication Data
Frankel, Bethenny.
    The skinnygirl dish : easy recipes for your naturally thin life /
Bethenny Frankel with Eve Adamson.
    p. cm.
    A Fireside book
    Includes index.
    1. Diet.   2. Nutrition.   3. Cookery.   I. Adamson, Eve.   II. Title.
    RA784.F674 2010
    641.5'63—dc22   2009035801

ISBN 978-1-4165-9799-5
ISBN 978-1-4391-0180-3 (ebook)

I dedicate this book to all of my Skinnygirls! You bought Naturally Thin, *you trusted the book, you trusted me, you lost the weight, and it changed your lives. I have read every single solitary testimonial and you in turn have changed my life forever. Trust this book, trust yourself, and continue your Skinnygirl journey.*

Contents

Introduction

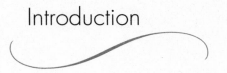

What's the Skinnygirl Dish?

have no food in this house. I'm standing in front of the open refrigerator and I don't have the slightest idea what to make for dinner. There is nothing to eat! I hate to cook. I don't know how to cook. I don't want to cook. I worked all day and I'm exhausted. If I cook, I'll have a huge mess to clean up. The last place I want to go right now is the supermarket. My kids are whining at me because they are hungry. I'm totally overwhelmed. I'm so uninspired. I don't have time to be healthy. Cooking is just too hard. It's too much to deal with. Maybe I'll just order a pizza. . . .

Stop right there, Skinnygirl! Calm down, breathe, and think this through. You *do* have food in the house, even if you don't immediately see a pre-made meal as you stare into the refrigerator. You *don't* have to fear, hate, or dread cooking. And you don't have to call the pizza guy.

In my first book, *Naturally Thin*, I showed you how to stop the food noise and begin listening to your food voice. In this book, I'll show you how to *stop the cooking noise* and listen to your inner chef. Cooking can be stressful if you make it stressful, but it doesn't have to be. Instead, you can learn to feed yourself well without stressing yourself out.

I don't have time to cook, either. I come home exhausted, too. Sometimes I do order a pizza, but I'll make it special. I'll order the whole-wheat crust (when that's an option) and make a big fresh Greek salad to go with it. Then I let myself really enjoy it. Most of the time, however, I make something. I wouldn't call it cooking as much as it is putting together things I already have in my refrigerator and my pantry. Get creative and the delicious results won't break the bank or make you feel as if you overate.

You have time to be healthy because it doesn't take very much time at all. That's the gist of this book: an end to the anxiety about what and how to eat when you have to cook for yourself and your family.

What to Eat

In *Naturally Thin*, I shared ten rules for unleashing your inner Skinnygirl and freeing yourself from a lifetime of dieting. As the *New York Times* best-seller list describes it, the book contains "rules and recipes for escaping the diet trap." That's exactly how I see it. Dieting is a trap, and it had me caught for many years. The point of that book was to set you free with new ideas for how to manage the food in your life.

If you've already read my previous book, you have the tools to be in control no matter how hazardous the situation may be, how stressful or inconvenient your schedule is, how hormonal you are, or how unusual your lifestyle might be. You can handle *any* pizza moment because you've been building a healthier relationship with food and you are well on your way to being naturally thin for life.

But the question remains: When you are tired, cranky, bored, uninspired, and just plain *hungry*, what are you going to eat? *Naturally Thin* brought you here. Now, *The Skinnygirl Dish* is the next step on your Skinnygirl journey.

I know from the many letters and e-mails I receive every day that a lot of you are still working on getting back in touch with your own hunger. I want to help you keep moving in the right direction, toward a realistic idea of what it means to eat like a naturally thin person. In this book, I'll walk you through my kitchen, my cooking philosophy, and the way I put a meal together. I promise you, none of it will be intimidating, difficult, time-consuming, or expensive. I just don't cook that way. Instead, I've tweaked my favorite comfort foods to make them more in tune with my Skinnygirl lifestyle, and I'll share those secrets with you. Most important, I'll show you *how* to cook—not just how to follow a recipe—so that you can stay inspired to steer clear of heavy habits and embrace thin thoughts every day.

The heart of this book is a new set of tools to teach you how to answer the question: "What am I going to eat?" No, I'm not going to tell you what to eat. If you read *Naturally Thin,* you know that's not what I do. What I will tell you is *how* to make something you will like in a way that works with your individual lifestyle. I want to give you the tools to cook *fearlessly* for yourself, taking risks, being creative, thinking for yourself, and never stressing out again about how to make dinner.

Food is important. Food is pleasure, comfort, community. Food is *delicious.* It's also one of the most powerful tools you have for building a healthy body and a calm mind. Food can make you strong or weak, energized or depleted, skinny or fat. What you eat can affect your hair, your skin, and your mood. It all depends on your choices. As the old saying goes, you are what you eat. You learned all that in *Naturally Thin.* For better or for worse, life isn't cookie-cutter. We plan and God laughs, as they say. You and I will continue to make mistakes occasionally—bad investments, regret, food noise, emotionality regarding food. I still wish I exercised a little more, drank a little less. We're all human. I don't pretend to be some perfect person with all the answers who is going to transform you into somebody you aren't.

Yet you and I are getting there and feeling freer than ever. Like yoga or anything else challenging, being naturally thin is a *practice.* You will never be perfect because nobody is perfect, but you are on the path and you are focused. I often give people this bit of business advice: You don't have to know exactly where you are going, as long as you are moving forward.

The Skinnygirl Dish will help you move forward. Throughout this book, I'll occasionally remind you of the ten secrets from *Naturally Thin,* but I'll include new rules I've learned since I wrote that book, as well as some ideas that didn't quite fit into that book's structure or that I thought would be too much information all at once.

I will also walk you through some of the things I make for myself, telling you how and why I chose to create those meals. There will be no intimidation in my kitchen, I swear to you! You will not find duck à l'orange or coq au vin or chateaubriand in this book because, frankly, those are not foods that I or any of my friends ever want to cook or eat at home. When you want some crazy foam mousse or shellacked salmon or beet puree, go visit an expensive fancy restaurant on your anniversary. You won't find those dishes here. I wouldn't even know how to start making them.

I am a natural foods chef. I went to a culinary school that specialized in food and healing with health as a priority, and I certainly can cook delicious food. However, I am not French trained. Bobby Flay would put me to shame with his knife skills and technical experience. Jean-Georges won't be calling me to give him cooking lessons anytime soon, and my plates don't look like pieces of art, even though I like to make them look attractive.

I specialize in figuring out how to make comfort food healthy. I'm talking about chicken pot pie and mashed sweet potatoes, baked ziti and red velvet cupcakes, and banana bread. I play around in my kitchen, taking all of my best friends' favorite foods that they are afraid to eat because they are too fattening and finding a way to make them good investments. Making low-fat guacamole and spinach artichoke dip that only tastes decadent is what I love. These are the foods that people crave, eat, then feel guilty about eating, but I think everybody should be able to enjoy the foods they love without guilt. Cooking should be accessible, tasty, healthy, and quick.

That's why this book is neither a cookbook nor a diet plan. It takes the best parts of both of those kinds of books and puts them together. Every single recipe in this book came from this situation: I was home. I was hungry. I looked in my kitchen to see what I had, and I made something out of it. I never once went to the store and bought every single ingredient for a recipe I wanted to make. This book is about using what you have and making it healthful and delicious. It will teach you how to cook the Skinnygirl way, built on a methodology you can trust. I don't care who you are or how bad a cook you think you are. If you can read, this book can teach you how to cook for yourself.

Your Kitchen, Your Wardrobe

In *Naturally Thin,* I compared your diet to your bank account. In *The Skinnygirl Dish,* I want to work from a new metaphor: *Food is like your wardrobe.* You all know what it's like to stand in front of your closet with the door hanging open and wonder why you have a closetful of clothes and nothing to wear, or why you hate everything you have and can't possibly wear any of it. Maybe you don't even get that far. Maybe you know what it's like to come home after a long day, lie down on the couch, and just dread getting up again and trying to figure out what to wear for an evening out.

Dinner can feel like a comparable situation as you stand in front of your refrigerator and think that you have absolutely nothing you can possibly eat or make or even begin to imagine you could pull out of there for dinner. Maybe you're lying on that same couch after work, thinking there is just no way you can get up and cook dinner.

This book is here to end all that.

My friends tell me that I should have a TV show called *What's in Your Kitchen* because I can go into anybody's kitchen when they say they have nothing to eat and find enough to make a delicious meal. I could probably do the same thing peeking into someone's closet and find them something to wear, but that's a different book. In this book, I'm going to show you how to work that magic in your kitchen.

To continue my clothing analogy, you need to know what classics to have on hand—the culinary versions of the black turtleneck, the crisp white shirt, the perfect jeans, the blazer, and the simple black dress. Then you need to venture out and be daring. Right now, as I write this, I'm wearing a pair of fuchsia patent leather pumps. An equivalent might be to dress up a simple bowl of brown rice with fresh herbs, or to bring a simple container of baby greens alive with dried cranberries or cherries and toasted sunflower seeds or almonds. It might mean you marinate a chicken breast or pork loin in a gourmet vinegar and some exotic herb. Accessorize your grains with things like olive oil, garlic, fresh herbs, pesto, sun-dried tomatoes, or pine nuts. Accessorize your protein basics with mustard, soy sauce, spices, and flavorful oils. Greens get dressed up with full-flavor grated cheese, nuts, dried fruits, and dressings. You'll find more complete lists in Chapter 2, but you get the idea.

This is how you make cooking exciting without making it complicated. Sometimes you take risks and sometimes you play it safe, but even when you wear the black turtleneck and the jeans, you can add flair by raiding your costume jewelry box or your makeup drawer or by putting on a really great watch. That's what I do when I get dressed and, equivalently, when I make food for myself at home. It's easy if you know how to put things together.

That's what this book will show you. If you were to ask me, "What are you going to eat?" this book would contain my answer. Like me, you will still dine out, go on vacation, go to sporting events, and face the occasional vending machine, minimart, or conference table full of doughnuts. When you do, you'll use the *Naturally Thin* tools to make smart investments. With this book, you can add more to your Skinnygirl arsenal so that you can confidently fill in the blanks when you are lucky enough to eat at home.

Every time I give you a recipe, I will provide variations and creative suggestions so that you can turn my ideas into years of options based on your own personal needs and desires. You can surprise your family night after night with simple changes and fresh variations. Variety is the new spice of your life, because with my recipes, you will always have choices.

That's another important part of this book: choice. This book is about my choices, but only for the purpose of assisting you with making your own choices. If I say I ate a steak salad, I don't want you blindly to run out and buy all the ingredients to make that exact steak salad. Instead, because you happen to have salmon left over from dinner last night, make a salmon salad. If you made chicken or ordered it in a restaurant, then a chicken salad version might be for you. It's your meal and your life, not mine. I want to see you get creative, even a little bit outside of your comfort zone. Think about what restaurants do to the foods they serve you. Consider the presentation and the interesting combinations of flavors. You can do that at home. Those creative ideas aren't just for restaurants. I'll help you. Just consider me your personal idea girl.

That brings me to the final reason for writing this book. I'm a pretty thrifty person and I hate to waste anything. I also try to live in an environmentally conscious way. Those concepts come into play specifically in this book as I talk about one of the primary ways I decide what to make for a meal: *using what I already have.*

Do you buy a new bag, lipstick, and dress every time you go out? Of course you don't. You look in your closet and you find what works. You can make it fresh and new without spending a dime by getting creative, and the same goes for food. If I have a take-out container of leftover steak and buttered baby peas, I'm not going to go out and buy a pork loin or chicken breast or a long list of exotic spices to make some recipe I saw in a magazine. I'm going to think about what I can do with that leftover steak and those peas. This is why I constantly rip out recipes from magazines and then *never use them.*

Maybe I'll stir-fry my leftovers with a little soy sauce and serve over rice with spices I already have in my cabinet. A chilled pea soup with half of a grilled steak and cheese sandwich on sourdough bread might be good, or maybe I'll put them both over fresh greens for a big salad with shredded carrots from my refrigerator and that last tomato. I might pick up a lemon or two for a fresh vinaigrette, but the gist of the meal comes from what's already in my kitchen. It's thriftier, and it's less wasteful, too. I hardly ever throw away food, and why should you?

So what are *you* going to make?

My goal for this book is to reenvision an old expression: I don't want to give you a fish. I want to teach you to fish. If I give you a fish, that's like giving you a diet, or a recipe. If I teach you to fish, I give you strategies for eating, or cooking, on your own. You learn to think for yourself so that you can handle any crisis, any situation, anything that comes your way. You'll know what to do, naturally.

Learning how to cook the Skinnygirl way means letting go a little and becoming open to inspiration and your own creative impulses. You start with recipes, but you don't let them imprison you. Use the knowledge in this book to learn how to "fish" and you'll be able to turn whatever you have in your refrigerator into a great meal that will keep your body slim and healthy and your discerning palate satisfied.

Confidence is key in this process. The more you learn about how to make good-investment food that tastes great, the easier it gets. You aren't going to start out making osso buco on the first day. Start simple. Or just stay simple. This is a simple book about simple, delicious comfort food and how to cook it well.

Beyond the Recipe

It may seem impossible to you right now, but the ultimate goal of this book is to set you free from the pages of a cookbook. Remember in high school when you would study and study for a test and then suddenly you just *knew* the information? Or think about learning to ride a bike or to swim. It's a struggle at first, but once you get it, you really *get it*. It becomes part of who you are, integrated into your consciousness. You just know how to do it.

This is what can happen to you with cooking. I think that recipes are a bit like kindergarten. You learn some basics, but then you eventually grow out of them and go out on your own. When you know *how* to cook, you won't need a recipe anymore.

This book *does* contain recipes, though, surrounded by stories about what I was doing when I decided to make the things I made. I'll show you how I did it, but I don't want you to stay chained to my concepts. This book is a Skinnygirl collection of ideas about how to stock your kitchen the same way you stock your closet, how to think like a chef, and how to make simple meals you can whip up on the go without feeling like you've compromised your healthy perspective or your budget.

I'll tell you all about my own kitchen, my must-have basics, the equipment I consider essential, and the things I really don't think you need at all. I don't spend a ton of money on food, and why should you? Good food doesn't have to cost a lot, take a lot of time to make, or contain ingredients that are impossible to find. Frankly, I shop more often at Costco and Trader Joe's than I shop at any expensive gourmet markets.

I've organized this book into three parts. Part One gives you the skinny—the basics you need to start feeling more confident in the kitchen, with or without a recipe. You'll learn how to cook, how to use what you have, and how to think like a chef. You'll get a peek into my kitchen, and I'll tell you what basics to stock and how to shop. I'll also share some of the cooking mistakes I've made in the past and how to avoid them.

Part Two is divided into six categories: breakfast, lunch, dinner, snacks, drinks (which include cocktails), and desserts. This part of the book contains recipes, stories, and tips about what I made, why, and how you can make these things into what *you* want to eat, according to what you have on hand.

Part Three consists of Skinnygirl Special Features, with chapters on entertaining (with recipes for amazing hors d'oeuvres), holidays, and recipes from some of my favorite chefs.

By the end of this book, I hope you will feel filled with confidence that you can always make a great meal, a tasty snack, or a delicious dessert; that you can handle any special occasion with confidence and flair; and that you actually don't mind getting up off that couch to make dinner. Because it's not hard. It's easy to cook like a Skinnygirl.

Part One

The Skinny

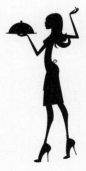

Chapter 1

How I Cook and How to Make It Yours

*R*ealizing that you can cook will be revolutionary. Cooking is easy, and I'm not saying this because I went to culinary school or have some innate gift. I don't mean cooking is easy for *me*. I mean cooking is easy for *you*.

People tend to overthink cooking, just like they overthink dieting. Even though you may not love to cook, you don't have to hate it. You just have to know how to do it.

I'm talking to all you people who really can't stand the idea of cooking. Yes, you people who can't bear the thought of getting up off the couch and making dinner after a long day of work. I'm a chef, and I don't always want to cook. I don't always want to get up off the couch, either, but we all need to eat, and going out every night is expensive. Cooking may seem overwhelming to you now, but it's really not hard at all, so forget the intimidation factor. Forget being overwhelmed. Forget that comment somebody made ten years ago about how you couldn't cook. That's done. It's over.

When you calm down and eliminate your cooking noise that tells you that you can't cook or that you hate to cook, you will find the space and the peace of mind to discover that you can make meals in no time. If you like to cook, you are already a step ahead of the game.

Sometimes I cook for celebrities, on the set or in their homes, and sometimes I think I shouldn't even get paid for it because the way I cook is so simple. Anyone can do it. Anyone. This book is not about multistep, labor-intensive cooking. It's about finding good ingredients in your own kitchen and putting them together for memorable Skinnygirl meals that take just a few minutes.

If you follow the advice and learn the basic concepts in this book, you will never have to buy another cookbook. Of course, you *can* buy another cookbook, but this is the last one you'll need. This is the book to set you free in your very own kitchen, to help you unleash your inner chef so that you will no longer be chained to the limitations of a recipe. My cookbooks have been sitting untouched for ten years.

I've always seen recipes as guidelines, not rules. A recipe is like a tour book of a city. You have it with you, but you don't necessarily use it. Sometimes you get an idea from it, but then you go your own way. If you want to follow the tour book, it can be fun and interesting, but when something beckons off the beaten path, you might want to go that way and have an adventure, take a risk. That's what chefs do, and you are about to become a Skinnygirl chef.

That's why I want to show you how to cook the food you want to cook, based on the ingredients you like and already have in your kitchen. *Use what you have.* On top of that, you'll cook food that is lightened up without sacrificing flavor. You'll learn to use the best ingredients where they count, and the easiest, quickest ingredients where they don't make that much of a difference—a variation of the *differential* concept from *Naturally Thin.* You'll learn when to splurge and when to hold back, and best of all, you'll learn to create variations on any theme according to what's exciting to you. You'll make your cooking personal and free it from the confines of what someone else is telling you to make.

That being said, I will give you recipes in this book, but they are both instructional and conversational rather than authoritarian. They are meant to show you how to think about cooking so that you won't need them anymore, except for reference. Every single recipe in this book came from using what I have in my kitchen. If I run out of stock, I use water. If I happen to have parsley, I use it instead of dill, or vice versa. That's why I made every recipe adaptable. You can make every recipe in this book at least five different ways, according to what you have. Use your creativity, and the variations will be truly endless.

When I graduated from culinary school and began cooking for people professionally, I looked at every cookbook I could get my hands on, stressing out over what to make. Now, I could throw them all away. Ninety percent of what I now know about cooking, I learned after going to cooking school. That gave me confidence in the kitchen, but now I put meals together in my own way.

What Cooking Is

Cooking is just getting food ready to eat. It isn't some mystical complicated process. You only need to master a few basic techniques and learn a few rules about ratios and ingredients, and you can make just about anything. When I want to make something new, I first look at a lot of recipes to get the basic elements, like how much chicken or flour or sweetener to use, then I put it together in a way that makes sense to me. You can do this, too. Then, if you choose to follow a recipe, fine. You'll be able to do it with confidence, knowing what you are doing. You'll even be able to improvise. Practice makes, maybe not perfect, but *better*.

When you don't have a recipe, you'll be just as capable of looking into your clean, organized, well-stocked refrigerator and your smartly furnished pantry to choose exactly what to make for a fabulous dinner with very little effort. That's how I cook, and that's how I want to teach you to cook, too.

In *Naturally Thin*, I talked about how food is not your best friend and not your enemy. In the same way, cooking is not your friend and cooking is not your enemy. It's just cooking, and when you let go of the emotionality, you set yourself free to have a little fun. When I cook, I like to experiment. I don't always use the most expensive ingredients. For lunch today, I made a simple soup out of frozen peas. Use what you have—take simple, basic food and make it special with interesting flavors such as fresh lemon juice, basil, or mint.

There are those people who always dress the same and look the same. Then there are those who dress with flair and take chances. You can be both. You can decide to go with the classics on some days, and on other days, you can bust out with an interesting spark. You'll be surprised by how many things go together when you get creative—basil in Chinese food, cherries on salad, arugula on a sandwich, a swirl of pesto in soup. It's harder to screw up than it is to succeed.

The more you embrace simple cooking and learn not to fear it, the more you will grow your relationship with food in your own kitchen. This will not only help you get a good Skinnygirl dinner on the table, but it will make eating to be naturally thin a lot easier, too. You'll control the variety in your own meals, as well as the quality of the ingredients, without ever having to get stressed out. You'll know exactly what's in your food, because you made it, and you'll know how to make it fun and exciting with basics and *wow*-factor items.

In *Naturally Thin*, I taught you how to balance your choices and *check yourself before you wreck yourself*, especially in restaurants and when out with friends. You can do all of those things at home, too. This book contains more than twice the number of recipes in *Naturally Thin*, so you can cook simple, delicious food made with fresh, healthful ingredients that are good investments. You'll get to eat more of what you love because the recipes in this book are customizable to your tastes, plus they are all good investments, with all the taste and a fraction of the fat and calories. That includes pasta, roasted chicken, vegetables that taste delicious, appetizers and party food, holiday food and desserts.

Your Kitchen, Your Closet

In the introduction to this book, I told you about my new favorite metaphor: Your kitchen is like your closet. If you know what it's like to stand in front of a closet full of clothes and realize you have nothing to wear, you probably also know what it's like to stand in front of a refrigerator full of food and realize you have nothing to eat. Let's talk about this a little bit more, because it's an important theme for this book.

Food and fashion have a lot in common. In many ways, the clothes we wear and the food we eat define us. But what to wear eludes many of us, and so does what to eat. That's because even though we know what we want to look like and what we should eat, even what we *want* to eat, there is often a gap between that knowledge and the actual construction of an easy, delicious meal. How do you get from point A to point B?

Let me give you another analogy. I've made a lot of fashion mistakes in my day. I've even made the worst-dressed list once, but I've learned from my mistakes, and what I've learned is that you have to know what to use and when to use it. Everything doesn't go with everything else. I'm not going to put basil on my cinnamon ice cream, and I'm not going to wear that seersucker jumpsuit . . . well, anywhere, ever again. You have to know what to wear for what events. You don't wear a cocktail dress to an MTV party. You wear something rock-and-roll. You learn those lessons the more you are out there. In the same way, the more you cook, the more you learn that basil is an excellent choice sprinkled on fresh ripe tomato slices with mozzarella cheese.

If you have dependable, high-quality classics you can rely on, you can then venture out and be daring with flavor accessories, the equivalent of great costume jewelry, red pumps, or an outrageous shade of lipstick. Dressing like that is easy, and cooking like that is easy, too.

Look, I'm no martyr. I am a housewife on TV, but even if I really was a housewife, do you know of one who makes fresh pasta or bakes bread every day? Cooking doesn't have to be so complicated. I always used to check my luggage on flights. Now I carry on my luggage, even for a two-week trip to Europe, because I've learned how to mix and match a few basic pieces to go anywhere. It's the same with cooking. It's the Garanimals approach— remember those kid clothes where you just matched the tags and any top would go with any bottom? When your kitchen has the right things, you learn how to put things together just like that. Ultimately, you will eat less because you will be more satisfied with your meals.

Sometimes it's fun to be the culinary hero and go the extra mile, but most of the time, that's not what I do. Most evenings aren't your wedding day or the most special night of your life. You just want food that tastes good. Very good. But it doesn't have to be a gourmet culinary creation.

I know you are busy, and I want to give you the ability to cook healthy meals that are easy but impressive and fulfilling. I want to start you out with recipes that you can trust, but even more important, I want you to feel confident than you can put together a meal all by yourself, without my help. The goal of this book is to help you learn how to trust yourself in the kitchen.

Making It Yours

In *Naturally Thin,* I told you that I was not going to tell you what to eat. Instead, I empowered you to listen to your food voice and discover what you really want to eat, not what some celebrity or diet guru tells you to eat. In *The Skinnygirl Dish*, I'm not going to tell you what to cook, either. I want to empower you to discover what *you* want to cook based on what you keep in your kitchen.

You can follow my recipes, of course. I recommend that you do, because they will help you learn about cooking. Then, if you keep your kitchen stocked with classics and accessories, you will have all the tools in place to make your own culinary creations. The recipes in this book are your launchpad, and from there, you can take off and make the food that you want to make, that you and your family will love. They will show you how to accessorize your meals the way you would accessorize a boring black dress to make it look exciting and fresh.

One of the reasons I always put so much emphasis on making food from your leftovers is because you already know you like your leftovers. You ordered the things you like when you were at the restaurant. When you bring home your leftovers, you have the opportunity to make that food into other foods you like because you have the basic items and skills you need.

Even when you don't have leftovers, how you shop will make your meals yours. I might buy a different kind of rice than you would buy, or you might prefer pasta. Some people like salads with Gorgonzola and toasted walnuts. I prefer pine nuts and Parmesan. What kind of salad person are you? I might focus more on steak and you might prefer salmon. Maybe you're a vegetarian and you are all about tofu. You can still make almost every recipe in this book, and more important, you will learn from this book how to make the food you love without the recipe, no matter what food you want to make. You don't have to stick with your preferences, either. The versatility of the recipes in this book will also allow you to push your own boundaries and experiment with tastes and ingredients you might not have dared to try before. Remember from *Naturally Thin* that *variety is the spice of life.*

Becoming a confident cook who isn't chained to a recipe is not just handy but empowering. It's all part of living the Skinnygirl life. People are attracted to good, natural, intuitive cooks. They trust someone who can produce delicious, healthy food without following a recipe to the letter. And while we're on the subject, and at least in my experience, the way to a man's heart really is through his stomach (just ask my fiancé), so gaining confidence in the kitchen can add a whole new element to your social life, too. But this book isn't about finding a man or winning friends or influencing people with your newfound cooking skills. In essence, *The Skinnygirl Dish* is a simple, sensible, straightforward, and budget-conscious plan for cooking, eating, and living the Skinnygirl life you learned to embrace from *Naturally Thin.*

About Safeties, Risks, and Happy Accidents

In this book, I'll often mention *safeties, risks,* and *happy accidents.* A safety is a trick or a technique that you know always works, or even something you know how to make that is always good. Safeties can be your signature dishes, your secret spices, your never-fail tools. They can be the recipes your kids beg you to make again and again, the ones your husband gets excited about, or just the ones you know will always make you feel better. Safeties are great to have in your repertoire, especially if you are entertaining and you can't risk making a mistake. Safeties are your ace in the hole.

But so are risks. Risks are the daring things you try when you are getting creative with your cooking. They might be new ingredients you found at a grocery store, or when visiting a foreign country or another city, or an inspiration you have while cooking that you think might really add something over-the-top-amazing to your meal. Sometimes risks turn into disasters. Your bright idea doesn't work. But so what? Now you know, and next time, you'll try something else.

Other times, risks result in happy accidents—when the result is more delicious or incredible than you dreamed it would be. Every mistake is a learning experience in the kitchen (and in life), and every risk has the potential to turn into something truly great. See Chapter 5 for some stories about my own cooking disasters, like when I used vanilla soy milk in my pasta carbonara. Do I have to tell you that was a bad, bad accident? That same day, when I mistakenly used vanilla soy milk for my cheesecake recipe, it was fantastic. You win some, you lose some.

Happy accidents are great. Once you start embracing them, you'll notice them in every aspect of your life. Did I think I would walk into a nightclub and end up marrying the guy who said, "Are you going to get that stick out of your ass?" No. I could have gone in there and met no one, but I took a risk, got out there, and there he was. Now I have a ring on my finger. Sometimes risks work and sometimes they don't, but where would you be if you never tried anything? In fact, my entire career has been a risk and a gamble . . . and I feel like I'm winning.

Even with the mistakes, I believe you will enjoy more successful meals than if you would have remained a slave to a cookbook full of recipes and never took any risks. They are worth the fun and the potential for happy accidents. When a risk does work, it can transform your everyday cooking into something really memorable and special. A really successful risk can then become a future safety.

What Is a Skinnygirl?

Before we jump into stocking your kitchen or making dinner, I want to go into a little more depth about the word *Skinnygirl*. In *Naturally Thin*, I gave you ten rules to live and eat by, and I'd like to remind you of them now, since I refer to them throughout this book. If you are living the Skinnygirl life, you may already have these memorized. They apply not just to eating but to cooking, too. Keeping these rules in mind no matter where you are—out at a restaurant or eating at home—will help keep you on track and headed in the right direction. Always remember:

1. Your diet is a bank account. Balance what you eat—types of foods and sizes of meals and snacks, good investments, and splurges—so that you never get too much of one thing.

2. You can have it all, just not all at once. When it comes to splurges, pick the one you want the most. You don't need to have it all at one meal. Do you want to splurge on the pasta, the bread, the wine, or the dessert? You can always make a different choice the next time.

3. Taste everything, eat nothing. When faced with a lot of decadent choices, just have a few bites of each. The sum total will equal a meal, but you won't have overindulged.

4. Pay attention. Notice when you are eating. Never eat while doing something else, because you won't get the satisfaction out of your food and you'll be more likely to overeat.

5. Downsize now. Enough with the huge portions. Just have a little of the good stuff and fill up on high-volume vegetables, soup, and grains.

6. Cancel your membership in the clean plate club. **Nobody is going to slap your hand with a ruler if you don't finish it all. Pay attention to how you feel. When you've had enough, *stop*, even if you leave just one bite.**

7. Check yourself before you wreck yourself. **Don't binge. The end. Don't do that to yourself ever again.**

8. Know thyself. **We all have our tendencies, our strengths, our weaknesses, our preferences. The more you know about yourself, the more successful you'll be at staying on track.**

9. Get real. **Real food is always a better investment than processed food.**

10. Good for you. **Do what's right for you, what's healthy for you, what's good for you. If you don't take care of yourself, you can't take care of anything else. Build a firm foundation of good health and self-care, and you can do anything.**

If you live by these rules, then you can eat anything you want to eat and cook any food you want to cook while staying or becoming naturally thin. You'll be a Skinnygirl as soon as you begin to see your food choices in light of these rules. Skinnygirl does not mean bone-thin. Only dogs like bones. Being a Skinnygirl doesn't mean you have to be a size 2 or 4. It might mean looking vibrant, healthy, beautiful, and curvy in a size 10 or 12 or 14 or whatever size you wear, and feeling good in it.

A Skinnygirl loves herself, lives her life to the fullest, and knows how to eat, drink, and be merry without fearing or obsessing over food. A Skinnygirl *owns her life*. She dresses to accentuate her best features rather than fearing or overexaggerating what she perceives as her flaws. She eats what she wants and stops when she knows she's had enough.

A Skinnygirl also likes, or can learn to like, cooking if it is effortless, stress-free, and she has all the ingredients right at her fingertips. Skinnygirls don't sweat it in the kitchen. Sometimes I dread cooking because of the mess, but over the years, I've figured out how to minimize that mess. Why cook with tons of pots and pans and procedures?

Embracing the Skinnygirl life is a process, so I don't expect you to be all the way there right now. I'm not even all the way there right now, but one of the things I have mastered is what food to keep in my house and how to turn those staples into delicious, easy meals and snacks that I can trust to make me feel nourished and energized but not bloated and guilty.

You don't have to be a hero in the kitchen. Instead, spend your energy on living a flirty, fun, interesting, exciting, *delicious* life that isn't *all* about the food. You can like to cook. You can enjoy sharing a drink with friends and learn how to mix one yourself at home. You don't have to be sweating over the stove, locked in the kitchen, or stuck behind the bar to do it, either. The recipes and techniques in this book will set you free to eat, play, and love your Skinnygirl life.

Chapter 2

Show Me Your Kitchen and I'll Show You Mine

The revolution begins at home, right in your own kitchen, and the first step is to get your kitchen ready for you. A chef's kitchen is clean, organized, and stocked with the classic ingredients and accessory items that a good culinary "wardrobe" requires. Yours can be just the same.

If your kitchen is messy and cluttered with no free counter space, if your refrigerator is overflowing and you don't even know what is inside half those containers, if your pantry is bare or (even worse) full of food items you don't like and will never eat, how can you expect to unleash your inner chef? That's like trying to get dressed when your closet is full of clothes you hate or that don't fit. If you can't even find the pair of shoes you need, you won't look put together. If you can't find the brown rice or the sea salt or the rest of that fresh cilantro you just know has to be in the back of the refrigerator somewhere, you won't just have a hard time cooking—you will *hate* cooking.

You need to get organized now. If you use something (like your toaster) every day, keep it close, not five miles away. Make the appliances and tools you use most the most accessible. You don't need a tool for every single task. You don't need tons of space or equipment, either. Just keep what you really use and get rid of the clutter. You can use a few good tools for all your cooking jobs. Just rinse them off and use them again and again, rather than getting ten different things dirty. Keep it simple. It's time to turn over a new leaf. Fix your kitchen and you'll fix your attitude about food. This chapter is about how to do that, so let's start by looking at my kitchen.

My Kitchen and Yours

Even though I'm a chef, my kitchen is definitely not full of a lot of different cooking appliances and gadgets. My food processor usually stays under the counter. I hardly ever use it. The same goes for my juicer. If I want fresh juice, I go to the health food store and get it. If you get an anxiety attack thinking about how cluttered your cabinets are, you are not alone. I have "stuff anxiety," too, and my solution is to edit, edit, edit. It's a work in progress.

I keep my kitchen tools in white flower pots from IKEA. I keep my knives on a magnet. I use a few basic things, and that's all I need. I don't have a spacious country kitchen, and although that would be nice, I don't need one. A big kitchen is just more kitchen to clean. I don't want a huge rack of pots hanging from the ceiling. My kitchen is a small but charming part of my apartment. It's open and bright and luckily has a window, but if it was piled with clutter or dirty dishes, I wouldn't love it. I wouldn't go in there. I keep my kitchen really clean and minimal, so I like to be in there. Step-by-step, I make little changes and additions so that it's more aesthetically pleasing. I take care of it.

Take a good hard look at your kitchen. What do you love? What do you hate? What's covering up your work space (i.e., your countertops)? What do you have two of, and do you really need two? What can you toss or give away? Do you have ten different pans, some of them burnt or scratched? Get rid of the damaged ones. Get rid of the broken spatulas, the splintered wooden spoons, and the chipped dishes. A minimalist kitchen equipped with a few good-quality, functional tools is the easiest kitchen to cook in and the easiest kitchen to clean.

A great kitchen doesn't have to be expensive, either. Mine certainly isn't. My refrigerator cost about $400, my stove $300, my dishwasher $200, and my microwave $100. My next place will probably have fancier appliances, but truthfully, my food has never suffered from being cooked using budget appliances. Maybe my oven isn't exactly the temperature it says (many aren't), but I know my oven and I know how to adjust what I'm cooking so that it will work. Even expensive ovens fluctuate in temperature, just like scales. If you know you are five pounds lighter on your home scale or two pounds heavier at the doctor's office, you know to make an adjustment in your head (although for my real opinion on weighing yourself all the time, see *Naturally Thin*). If you know your oven runs a little hot or a little cold, you will learn to make those adjustments in your head when you cook. Or, play it safe and just buy an oven thermometer.

The same goes for my kitchen tools. My nonstick pans are from Costco, and I can tell they're probably made at the same factory as the fancier brands. *Consumer Reports* ranked my Costco pans above some well-known name brands. They do the job I need them to do. They aren't those cheap nonstick pans you can scratch with a plastic fork. It's worth investing in *high-quality* nonstick cookware, but even so, my pans cost me about $149 for the whole set, which isn't all that expensive considering how much I use them. I also have some Le Creuset pans, but truthfully, I find them bulky and difficult to pick up. Sometimes they are the perfect thing, but they aren't necessarily for every day.

Every kitchen needs a refrigerator, an oven, and a stove. You can probably get by without a microwave and a dishwasher, although they make cooking and cleanup a lot faster and easier. You also need some basic tools of the trade, which I'll explain in the next section. Just as important, you have to like your kitchen. Brighten it up with flowers or photographs you love. Paint it a great color. Change the hardware on the cabinets. These are all quick, easy, economical ways to make your kitchen more pleasant. When you have the time and the money, you can always do things like put

IS NONSTICK COOKWARE SAFE?

You may be wary of using nonstick cookware because you've heard it is made with chemicals that might end up in your food or might be dangerous to the environment. You know what? Maybe that's true. I don't know. I'm not a doctor or a scientist, but I hear about hot oil releasing carcinogens, and you have to use a lot more hot oil when you aren't using a nonstick pan. It's a trade-off. You can't do everything perfectly all the time, so do what you can, when you can, and weigh your options. To me, nonstick pans are well worth their many benefits—they are easier to use, easier to clean, and inexpensive. I'd love to live in an all-organic world, but what are you going to do—stay home and never eat and hide in the closet? Pick your battles and give yourself a break. In my life, high-quality nonstick cookware works.

in new cabinet fronts, countertops, and flooring, but don't worry about that now. The point is to make little tweaks to help lure you into your kitchen. It could become your favorite room in the house.

One of the most important ways I keep my kitchen pleasant is by editing. I can't emphasize this enough: it's very important to keep your refrigerator and cabinets clean and organized, just like your closet should be. Get rid of everything you don't use! I don't just mean burnt pans and old tools. I mean that jar of peppers that you are never going to finish, that expired cream cheese, those almost-slimy herbs. Better yet, use the herbs before they get slimy. Chop them up and mix them with brown rice or pasta. Once every week or two, go through every shelf of your refrigerator and pantry and throw away the things you know you aren't going to use. Just get them out of there, even if it means you have hardly anything left. Wipe down the shelves and arrange what's left with the labels facing forward so that you can see what you have. This isn't being obsessive. It's just being organized. If you aren't already in this habit, you have no idea how much easier and more pleasant it will make your kitchen experience.

If your kitchen is a real mess, don't feel like you have to do everything at once. I don't want you to feel overwhelmed, ever. Just tackle one shelf of your refrigerator or one cabinet. What's still good? What will you eat? If you like it, how could you use it in the next day or two? If you don't like it, out it goes. Be ruthless. When you get rid of the junk, you can actually see what you have to work with. Life is too short and food is too good to be wasted. Respect your kitchen and the food you keep in it, and your cooking skills will automatically improve. When you clear out the junk, it's like you've dropped ten pounds. You'll feel lighter and cleaner and better about yourself and your life. You might even start doing the same thing to your bedroom, living room, the cabinet under the bathroom sink. Editing is addictive because it has such a big payoff. You might as well start now. Just do one refrigerator shelf. Clean it off and wipe it down. Go ahead, I'll wait.

Tools You Can Use

Now that you are moving in the right direction, organizing your kitchen so that you like to be in it and you actually have room to cook there, let's talk about the basic tools you can use to make cooking as easy as possible.

Having the right tools in your kitchen is like having the right pieces in your wardrobe. You aren't going to buy them all at once. You will build your kitchen wardrobe over time. If you don't have a roasting pan, for example, don't go out and buy one until you are ready to roast a chicken or a turkey. Then the occasion calls for the investment. I'm not going to recommend that you spend hundreds of dollars on high-end gourmet cooking equipment, either. Personally, I rely heavily on just a few key tools, all of which you can buy inexpensively at almost any store that carries pots, pans, and utensils. I find a lot of brand-new items on eBay.

The first thing that comes to mind when I think about the tools I use the most is my immersion blender. I have a regular blender, but I hardly ever use it, and I don't bother to get my food processor out very often. And by that, I mean never.

I also rely on strong rubber spatulas, cutting boards, my reasonably priced knives, a microplane, liquid and dry measuring cups, a fine-mesh strainer, plastic storage containers, mixing bowls, measuring spoons, and a grater. Occasionally I use twine to tie chicken legs together, but right now I don't have any in my kitchen. The next time I roast a chicken, I'll get some. Sometimes I use a basting brush to put a light coating of oil or butter on things (whether it's a roast chicken or bruschetta), kitchen shears, and various wooden spoons and plastic spatulas for nonstick pans.

A set of solid nonstick cookware, including a large skillet with a lid, will become an invaluable part of your Skinnygirl kitchen. You'll use these pans again and again. To help them last, use wooden or nonstick utensils with them, never metal. Treat nonstick pans gently and never wash them with soap. Use only water and a plastic scrub brush, and they will last a long time. When the coating finally starts to wear off, just replace the pot or pan. I use my large nonstick skillet at least several times each week and daily when I'm developing recipes. The lid is essential! If you can find a skillet that can also go straight into the oven (it will have to have an oven-proof handle), the extra cost will pay off in convenience, especially when you only have to wash one pan instead of a skillet and a casserole dish.

To help you get organized, here is a list of what I consider essentials and also those things you might want to buy when the occasion calls for it. You probably already have a lot of these things in your kitchen:

Essential Items

- Quality nonstick cookware: small and medium saucepans, a large soup pot or Dutch oven, a small skillet, and a large skillet with a lid. Ovenproof is preferable.
- Nonstick baking pans: at least one baking sheet, two 9-inch cake pans, one square cake pan, one 9 × 13-inch baking pan, muffin/cupcake tins (12-cup tin or two 6-cup tins), a pie plate, and a regular-size loaf pan (9 inches). A release pan (springform pan) is also handy, especially if you don't like turning cakes out onto a plate. It's great for cheesecake, too. It has a side that unbuckles from the base.

- A set of mixing bowls in small, medium, and large.
- A few strong, heatproof rubber spatulas. I never use wooden spoons because I think rubber spatulas do everything wooden spoons can do and more.
- Two cutting boards, or just one: use one for meat and one for vegetables, or use one side for meat and the other for vegetables (label them with a permanent marker). Plastic is easiest to clean. (I use small, inexpensive wooden cutting boards for serving cheese at parties, but not for cutting, because I think bacteria gets into the wood.)
- Sharp knives. A chef's knife, a small paring knife, and a serrated knife for cutting bread and tomatoes is all you need. A sharpening stone or roller will keep your knives sharp. Just be careful not to cut yourself.
- A plastic scrub brush for cleaning nonstick cookware.
- An immersion blender with a regular blender attachment and a chopper attachment.
- A microplane: better than a grater for hard cheese, chocolate, citrus peel, and gingerroot. You get a lot of flavor with just a very fine grating.
- A regular or box grater, when you want a larger grating than you can get from a microplane. It's great for softer cheeses and vegetables like carrots, beets, and potatoes. The one I have is a box with the grating surface on top so that the cheese or vegetables fall into the container. It has a cover for storage and comes from IKEA.
- Measuring cups: a set of liquid cups in 1-, 2-, and 4-cup sizes, and a set of dry in ¼-, ⅓-, ½-, and 1-cup sizes.
- Measuring spoons: ¼-, ½-, and 1-teaspoon sizes, plus 1 tablespoon.
- Ice-cream scoops in a few different sizes. I use these constantly, not just for ice cream but for portioning out cookie dough, muffin batter, hamburger meat, crab cakes, and a million other things.
- A colander, for draining pasta and washing salad greens.
- Wooden skewers for testing baked goods when you don't have a toothpick, and for grilling (always soak wooden skewers in water be-

fore grilling so that they don't burn). You can also make fruit skewers (like the Rainbow Fruit Skewers in my first book).

- Toothpicks for testing baked goods for doneness.
- Individual ramekins. These ovenproof ceramic or glass bowls are great for cooking or serving things like ice cream. They are inexpensive, and I use mine constantly. They are the perfect size to help you control your portions.
- Tongs with rubber bottoms so that you don't scratch your nonstick pans.
- A fine-mesh strainer.
- A sifter, to lighten and aerate dry ingredients when you are baking.
- A whisk. Look for one that won't scratch your nonstick pans.
- A basting brush. Get a heatproof one so that the bristles don't melt when you baste a hot chicken.
- Kitchen shears. Indispensable.
- Butcher paper or parchment paper and aluminum foil, to make baking pans nonstick and to keep them clean.
- Plastic storage containers for saving leftovers.

Optional Items

- A mortar and pestle: nice for grinding rather than blending spices.
- A splatter screen, which can be helpful when you are sautéing.
- Kitchen twine, when you need it.
- A blender, if you like to make fruity frozen drinks like margaritas or if you are a smoothie person, but if your immersion blender has a blender attachment, you don't need this.
- A juicer: nice if you like to squeeze your own juice. I rarely have time to do that, and if I need lime or lemon juice for a drink, I usually just squeeze it by hand.
- A salad spinner. I would love to have one but I don't want to use up the space to store it, so I wash and dry my greens the hard way, in a colander.

- A mallet: good for pounding meat if you want to make it thinner, which some recipes call for.
- A larger roasting pan, with or without a rack, for when you want to cook a large chicken, turkey, or roast that won't fit in a 9 × 13-inch baking pan. I only use mine during the holidays.
- Mini muffin pans.
- An 8-cup glass measuring cup.
- A really large salad bowl if you serve a lot of people and need to make more salad than you can easily toss in a large mixing bowl.
- See Chapter 11 for information on what tools to have for a home bar, if you like to mix your own drinks.

Classics

Now let's talk about the food you will want to keep in your house most of the time. These items are like your classic wardrobe pieces that you rely on regularly to keep you put together. With these classics, you will always have something to eat that you can "dress up" with accessory or exotic items. Foods in some categories, such as seasonal vegetables, can be bought according to what looks good and what is available.

When you've finally cleared out and cleaned up your refrigerator, cabinets, pantry, and every other place you keep food, you'll know exactly what you have right now. Compare your current inventory with these lists of classics, then add what you don't have to your kitchen according to what makes sense for you.

You don't have to buy every item on these lists. In fact, I encourage you *not* to do that. Make it your own—stock the basics you like. If I say turkey and you prefer chicken or tofu, go with that. If I say Dijon mustard and you like yellow, stock what you prefer. You'll probably already have a lot of these things. If the list of things you don't have looks daunting, don't worry about doing this all at once. It can be a gradual process, just like cleaning and organizing and acquiring the tools you need.

Eventually, if you aim to have all these classics in your kitchen, you'll never again be stuck with nothing to eat.

If you really like and regularly eat something that is not listed here, of course you will keep it in your kitchen! Maybe it's tempeh or turkey ham, veggie hot dogs or low-fat pudding cups, or whatever. These are lists of what I consider classics. I want you to make them *your* lists, so don't consider these to be written in stone:

THE ESSENTIAL SIX

If I was limited to six and only six items that I always keep in my kitchen to accessorize meats, grains, and vegetables, I would choose these, which my kitchen is never without:

1. Olive oil
2. Lemons
3. Parsley

4. Garlic
5. Salt
6. Pepper

Your Refrigerator

This is where you keep your meat, dairy, and produce, as well as any shelf-stable condiments after you open them. I also keep opened bags of oatmeal, nuts, grains, cereal, and flour in the refrigerator to keep them fresher longer. If you keep these things in your cabinets, frankly, you could get weevils in them, and then you will throw up.

Proteins and Dairy

You can always try different cheeses, dried meats, or exotic kinds of milk, but these are the classic culinary wardrobe items to have on hand in your refrigerator when you need protein:

- Cheese, hard/soft. I usually have blue cheese, feta cheese, Parmesan, and soy cheese slices in my refrigerator. Include a crumbly cheese for salads, a hard cheese for grating, and a cheese you would want to use on a sandwich. Shredded cheese spoils more quickly, so I prefer to shred my own cheese from blocks or wedges, using a simple box grater. It tastes fresher. I also keep low-fat versions of cottage cheese, cream cheese, and sour cream on hand. You may only need to buy these as you need them, depending on your preference. Use nondairy if you prefer them. Or skip the cheese altogether.

- Yogurt. I like plain Greek yogurt made by Fage. Or, keep soy yogurt. It's great for snacks and for use in many recipes. Plain is more versatile because you can use it in savory cooking or add fruit, nuts, and sweetener to it for a snack.

- Eggs. I like the real thing, but back when I used to live in Fat-Free Land, I ate egg substitutes all the time, and I thought they were okay. Now that I am a convert to real food, I think they taste like yellow, egg-textured water. It's certainly up to you, but egg substitutes are highly processed. I have nothing at all against real egg whites in a carton, however. These are a good addition to your refrigerator, if you prefer them to whole eggs. Get the kind that contain just real egg whites, nothing else.

- Milk: low-fat, skim, soy, almond, rice, coconut, hazelnut, and so forth, in plain, vanilla, and chocolate—whatever kinds you like and use.

- Tofu, if you like it. The most versatile is the extra firm, but if you don't eat eggs, also keep silken tofu around, as it makes a good egg substitute for baking. The extra firm typically comes in a tub with water and the silken kind is usually vacuum packed.

- Bacon: turkey or veggie. This is great for flavoring a lot of things. You only need a little. If you don't have this around all the time, that's certainly fine, but I tend to keep it around.

- Turkey breast meat (sliced), or, if you prefer some other sliced meat, go with that. This is for quick sandwiches.

Fruits and Vegetables

There are so many exotic, interesting, fiber-rich, vitamin-rich fruits and vegetables out there that are fun to try when they are in season. However, at any given time I always have at least a few of the following in my refrigerator:

- Leafy greens. I usually have either arugula, baby spinach, or some kind of mesclun mix, but choose whatever you like for salads.
- Some type of greens for cooking: kale, chard, collards, beet greens, and so forth.
- Aromatics: onions (yellow, red, and/or white), leeks, or shallots; scallions; garlic; ginger.
- Vegetables for salads, such as carrots; celery; corn; and pear, grape, or cherry tomatoes.
- Celery.
- Some kind of potato: russet, red, gold, fingerling, or sweet.
- Fresh herbs. Don't buy too many at once, but it's always nice to have some fresh parsley or cilantro on hand, plus other favorite herbs.
- Seasonal assorted vegetables for roasting or sautéing: just one or two of whatever looks good, such as peas, asparagus, zucchini, bell peppers, corn on the cob, beets, or eggplant. These are great for mixing with rice for a snack or a light lunch.
- Apples: good for a quick snack.
- Lemons or limes, for flavoring almost anything.
- Assorted seasonal fruit, when it looks good: pears, peaches, plums, melons, grapefruits, fresh berries, oranges, tangerines, and so on.

Miscellaneous

A few other things that belong in every Skinnygirl's refrigerator:

- Bread, especially whole grain or sprouted grain. I like flatbread, pita, and Pepperidge Farm Deli Flats, which are just 100 calories each.
- Butter or vegan/soy margarine (the kind with no trans fat).
- Opened condiments, jarred foods, and, of course, leftovers.

Your Freezer

The freezer is where you keep more perishable items so that you always have them when you need them but don't necessarily have to worry about eating them up within a few days. I like to freeze individual containers of leftovers for quick meals. Of course, this is where you will also keep absolute essentials like ice cream. Here is what is almost always in my freezer:

Sweet Condiments

- Fruit-only jams or preserves. Choose a few you like, such as strawberry, peach, raspberry, or orange marmalade.
- Natural liquid sweetener you like, such as honey, maple syrup (real, not artificial), or agave nectar.

Nuts, Seeds, and Dried Fruits

- Nuts: one or two kinds, like slivered almonds, walnuts, cashews, pecans, macadamia nuts, or peanuts.
- Pine nuts.
- Seeds: one or two kinds, like sunflower, pumpkin, sesame, or poppyseeds.
- Nut butters: peanut, almond, or other.
- Dried fruit: one or two kinds, like raisins, apricots, cranberries, cherries, blueberries, or prunes. Yes, prunes. No one is mad at prunes.

Baking Ingredients

- Baking powder.
- Baking soda.
- Chocolate chips. I like miniature ones because I use fewer.
- Cocoa powder, unsweetened.
- Confectioners' sugar. I always use raw sugar unless I need confectioners' sugar (also called powdered sugar) for something like frosting. I've never seen raw confectioners' sugar, so I get the standard kind.
- Flavored extracts: vanilla and almond, plus others you like. Companies like Watkins make a lot of interesting ones.
- Shredded coconut, if you like it.
- Raw sugar, Sucanat, or turbinado sugar (like Florida Crystals).

Accessories

Once you've got the basics, you've always got something to eat, but since variety is the spice of life, you can add accessory items to your refrigerator, freezer, and pantry to keep things interesting and your cooking exciting. These are your scarves, your jewelry, your shoes—the things that give your classics flair.

You won't want to have all of these all the time. Don't be intimidated. In fact, this is just a selection from the great universe of foods out there. Try one or two every time you go to the store and see how you can work the new item into your cooking, or try things *you* find that look interesting to you, the way you would work a new necklace or scarf into an outfit. Be daring in your own way. These items are purely suggestions, but they are great to have on hand for splurges, dares, and culinary risk taking.

- Black sesame seeds. They have a bigger visual impact than regular sesame seeds but a similar taste. Try them on salmon, chicken, tofu, shrimp, and Asian salads.
- Coconut oil.
- Fish sauce: great for Thai and other Asian dishes.
- Flax meal or flaxseed, which you can grind into meal to add fiber and nutrients to oatmeal or baked goods.
- Hoisin sauce: a delicious sauce in Asian cuisine.
- Lemongrass: called for in many Asian recipes.
- Light coconut milk, especially if you like piña coladas and Indian and Thai food.
- Other extracts. Vanilla and almond are essential, but if you also keep a variety of extracts in flavors you like, such as coconut, mint, lemon, maple, banana, and rum, you'll have a lot of flexibility in baking. One cheesecake recipe can become twenty different cheesecakes if you use a different extract in each one.
- Pumpkin puree: great for low-fat baking.

HERBS, SPICES, AND SEASONINGS

Dried spices have a long shelf life, but not so long that you can keep them for years. They will lose potency and get dusty tasting. Smell your herbs and spices, or compare fresh with old, to get a sense of the difference. Throw out herbs and spices that have lost their fragrance. That being said, most people keep their herbs and spices forever so if they still smell okay, keep them.

Dried herbs have a different flavor, but sometimes they are just more convenient, so go ahead and use them as an alternative to fresh, keeping in mind that dried herbs have a deeper, more intense flavor. Here are some suggestions based on what I usually have in my kitchen:

- Basil
- Bay leaves
- Chili powder
- Coriander
- Cumin
- Curry powder
- Garlic salt
- Kosher salt or sea salt
- Mustard powder
- Oregano
- Paprika
- Parsley
- Pepper in a grinder (I use Kirkland from Costco)
- Rosemary
- Sage
- Spike seasoning (my secret weapon)
- Tarragon
- Thyme

- Saffron threads.
- Smoked paprika.
- Steak sauce (such as A.1.).
- Stevia: a natural herb sweetener some people like to use instead of sugar.
- Thai curry paste.
- Unusual or seasonal fruits and vegetables: guava, kiwi, breadfruit, papaya, and so on.
- Vanilla beans.
- Wheat germ.

Choosing the foods to stock your kitchen shouldn't feel like a chore—it should be fun. This is your game. Play it with enthusiasm and style, and it will show when you cook with the ingredients you've purchased and stored in your clean, organized kitchen.

Chapter 3

The Skinnygirl Chef's Essential Kitchen Rules

You don't wear white after Labor Day (or you do, but *on purpose*). You don't wear colors that don't look good on you or clothes that don't fit. You don't mix too many accessories into one outfit, but you do develop a unique style that works for you. Rules for dressing are a lot like rules for cooking. Know what they are before you decide to break them, but ultimately, develop your own style.

You already know I don't believe in diets, but I do believe in eating guidelines. I don't believe in hard-and-fast fashion rules, either, but I do believe in having some boundaries and knowing what you will and won't wear, and how you will and won't wear it. In the same way, I don't believe in recipes, but I do believe in a few essential kitchen rules. In this chapter, I'll share them with you because these are the rules that will *take the pressure off*. I want you to quit feeling stressed out and overwhelmed because you have to find something to make for dinner. Knowing the rules that work for you are what make cooking *easy*.

In *Naturally Thin,* I told you that I wasn't going to tell you what to eat.

Instead, I showed you *how* to eat—how to eliminate your food noise and listen to your food voice, how to make good investments by balancing your diet like a bank account, and how to eat any food you really want without overdoing it or feeling guilty. I gave you ten rules to free you from dieting anxiety. In this chapter, I'll give you the Skinnygirl chef's ten essential kitchen rules that will free you from your cooking anxiety.

Rule 1: Don't Be a Hero

Cooking can be difficult or easy. I opt for easy, unless easy seriously compromises the result. If cooking is stressful, maybe you are trying to be a hero. Most of the time, the easier option is just fine, and getting permission to take the easy road can feel like a huge weight being lifted off your shoulders.

Sometimes you just don't feel like washing your hair. So don't. Wear a ponytail or a headband. Sometimes a short cut is well worth the time and effort it will save you. It's the same with cooking. When you just want to get a good meal on the table fast, go easy on yourself. It's such a relief. You aren't running a gourmet restaurant, so don't be afraid to cut corners.

If you pressure yourself to do everything perfectly when you are cooking and then don't ever want to cook because of the pressure, *adopting this attitude can change your life*! I'm a perfectionist, too, but something's gotta give. I like to look really nice for a red carpet event or if I'm being photographed, I'll go all out. Otherwise, I'm just trying not to look like a slob. I just want to look nice. This is how I see everyday cooking. You can go all out for the big event if you really want to, but most meals just need to be good. They don't need to be the best meal you ever had in your life.

I will always let you know when an extra step is really worth the trouble, but believe me, I am a chef and I take the easiest road. I don't make my own stock; I don't always roll out a handmade piecrust.

Buying premade doesn't mean settling for low quality. The food you buy should be good and worth your money. For example, I almost always buy premade pesto, but I buy the fresh refrigerated bright green kind. I wouldn't touch the brown, shelf-stable kind in a jar. The same goes for tapenade, hummus, and tomato sauce—when I don't have time to make my own (even though these are all really easy to make), I find good fresh versions at the store or deli and doctor them with fresh herbs.

I think vegetable and chicken broth in a box tastes just fine, but think beyond the box. If your favorite Chinese restaurant or Jewish deli makes an amazing chicken or vegetable stock, ask if you can buy some. Most gourmet markets also have chef-prepared stock you can buy. Take it home, put it in the freezer, and then quit complaining. Now you have great stock that someone else made for you. If your favorite Italian restaurant has a great tomato sauce or pizza dough, ask if you can buy some of that. That being said, if you have lobster shells or a chicken carcass and a free Sunday and you want to try your hand at making homemade stock, go for it.

I don't own a restaurant. I have a lot of things to do every day besides cook, and you do, too. If you find good brands or versions of basic ingredients that taste good, you won't ever have to think about how you might try to make them at home unless you decide you *want* to try to make them at home.

Do you remember the concept of the *differential* that I talked about in *Naturally Thin?* In that book, I used the term to distinguish between two food choices and how to decide which one to eat. Just in case you need a refresher, think about veggie or turkey chili versus chili con carne with beef. If you like the veggie or turkey chili just about as much as the beef chili, then the *differential* is nothing. In that case, choose the better investment— the veggie or turkey chili. Now, compare a New York strip steak to a plain chicken breast. If you love the steak way more than the chicken (like I do), then the *differential* is huge. In that case, choose the steak, but enjoy just enough to get the experience, knowing it's a pretty high-fat food choice and not a great investment.

The point is that when the *differential* is small, choose the better investment. When the *differential* is big, don't deny yourself what you really want.

In this book, the *differential* comes into play in a slightly different way. If you think (like I do) that chicken broth in a box tastes perfectly fine, then why would you spend hours nursing along a homemade stock with a thousand ingredients you don't even have in your kitchen, especially if it's just one part of something else? If you are making homemade chicken soup, then sure, go for that stock. Otherwise, do you want to mess up your kitchen that much? Do you want to spend all that money? Do you really have time to hunt down all the fresh herbs for a bouquet garni? Do you even know what a bouquet garni is? Who cares? (But in case you just have to know, it's a combination of herbs bundled together in cheesecloth and dropped into stock or some other typically French dish while it cooks. You fish it out before serving.) In general, these are some guidelines for where it really does pay to take the easy way out:

- Use nonstick cookware instead of stainless steel. Maybe you've heard that all the really great chefs use stainless steel. Don't be a hero. If you don't want to cook with stainless steel, just buy a good set of nonstick cookware. You'll be able to clean it in seconds. I don't use stainless steel as often because you have to use a lot of oil. It's great to have experience with a stainless steel pan, so go ahead and use one when and if you want to. I'm just saying that I usually rely on my nonstick cookware for daily cooking chores. If you could care less about stainless steel, that's fine, too. Nonstick cookware is all the cookware a Skinnygirl really needs.

- Use a good boxed broth instead of homemade stock. I already talked about this, but I'd like to add that I never make homemade stock. Never. Every chef I know will have less respect for me, but I don't care. If you do make a beautiful Bobby Flay–style stock, your soup will taste a little bit better, but in my opinion, that doesn't outweigh how annoying it is to make a stock and how much it will mess up your kitchen. A good French-style stock has a lot of steps, and when I see fifty steps in any recipe, I get anxious. I promise you that no recipe in this book will have multiple steps or sections or parts. It's more important for me to be minimalist and keep it simple. By the way, for maximum flavor in any savory recipe, substitute broth for water.

- **Use good jarred or canned tomato sauce if you must.** The truth is that it takes five minutes to make homemade tomato sauce. It's easy. However, if you don't want to make it, then don't. Good tomato sauce in a jar is just fine. Tomato paste in a can or a tube is fine, too. Canned fire-roasted tomatoes—especially when tomatoes aren't in season and the so-called fresh tomatoes in the supermarket taste like nothing—are perfectly acceptable and even delicious. I'm not talking about cheap sugary spaghetti sauce. Buy good imported or fire-roasted tomatoes, particularly organic ones. Even when tomatoes are in season, if you don't feel like chopping them, use good canned tomatoes instead. The only time that fresh tomatoes really matter is when you are going to eat them raw, like in a salad or chopped with fresh herbs on bruschetta.

- **Buy hummus, tapenade, pesto, and salsa . . . unless you really want to make them.** Hummus, tapenade, pesto, and salsa aren't really all that hard to make from scratch. If you want to try making them, go ahead. But if you don't want to drag out your food processor or your blender or you don't feel like chopping a bunch of vegetables, you can buy really tasty versions of these items in the store. Maybe you've read that you can make your own pesto and freeze it in ice cube trays so that it is convenient. I have never met anybody who actually does that. It's easier to buy a fresh refrigerated version if you can find one you like. Whenever I buy anything premade, I always doctor the product with fresh ingredients and it becomes my own.

- **You don't have to bake bread.** Unless you love to bake bread, why go through the hassle? I certainly don't have time to bake bread and I don't want a giant bread machine taking up valuable real estate in my kitchen. Baking bread can be time-consuming and strenuous, and you have to deal with that whole yeast thing—is it alive, is it dead? Forget about it. You can get good freshly baked bread all over the place. Find a baker you trust at a grocery store or a bakery and buy your bread there. Put a loaf in the oven for a few minutes to make the crust crispy and spend your time making fancy butter instead. Add some pesto or tapenade to butter and everyone will be impressed. The same goes for dinner rolls, and pasta. Do you really want to make those from scratch? Me neither.

WHAT THE DOCTOR ORDERED

Add your own personal touch to store-bought dips and spreads so that they taste unique, fresh, and interesting. Try these doctoring tips:

- Add flavorful ingredients such as basil, lemon zest, and toasted pine nuts to store-bought hummus.
- Liven up the taste of tapenade with some chopped fresh parsley or other fresh herbs you have on hand.
- Brighten store-bought pesto with chopped fresh basil and an extra squeeze of fresh lemon juice.
- Give store-bought salsa more zip with a squeeze of fresh lime or lemon juice and some chopped fresh cilantro or parsley.

Rule 2: Use What You Have

I'll talk about how to implement this rule in Chapter 4 and throughout this book, but the basic point is that if your kitchen is well stocked, you can always find something to eat and you can also find substitutes for any ingredient you are missing. Recently, I wanted to make jerk chicken, and one of the key ingredients in this dish is Scotch bonnet peppers. However, my assistant forgot to buy the Scotch bonnet peppers. I guessed that a tablespoon of crushed red peppers would be about right for a substitute, and it worked. I took a risk, and it paid off. Again, it's like fashion: You don't buy a whole outfit every time you go out. You use what you have, but you figure out how to put it together in a fresh way.

I never follow recipes to the letter, and I'm certainly not going to go out and buy every single ingredient in a recipe when I have things at home that are close enough. For example, you can replace leeks with onions or scallions, dried herbs with fresh, basil with oregano, broccoli with zucchini, chicken with fish. (Recently, I read about a scallion recall. Use chives instead.) Every change you make will change the result a bit, but that doesn't mean the dish won't still be good. It will just be different and sometimes it will be a happy accident. Taking chances can be liberating. Besides, give ten chefs the same recipe and they'll come out with ten different dishes. Chefs hate to be pinned down to the confines of a recipe (I know I do), so why shouldn't you be similarly creative . . . and *thrifty* . . . by using up the food you already paid for instead of buying more? Use what you have and you'll be forced to be more creative with your cooking. You might also get some lessons about what works and what doesn't. (See Chapter 5 for some hilarious stories about recipes I made that didn't work out the way I planned.)

Rule 3: Something's Got to Give

Whenever I renovate a recipe, my main goal is to make comfort food a better investment without sacrificing taste. Sometimes it works and sometimes my attempts are dismal failures, but I keep trying different approaches. What I've realized after years of overhauling recipes is that when you are improving a recipe and you want it to taste good, something's got to give.

You can't strip off every single accessory or go out in your bathrobe. You have to splurge somewhere—the well-cut jeans, the nice watch, the up-do. In the same way, you can't take out all the fat, all the sugar, all the meat, or all the flour from a dish without sacrificing taste, and I'm just not willing to do that. I don't want to eat food that tastes bland, fake, and gluey, and you don't, either. *It has to taste good.* Take out what doesn't matter that much and leave a little of the good stuff so that the result is still satisfying. The more you practice this, the more you learn about what you can sacrifice without missing it.

It's all about the differential. You cut fat and calories where it won't affect the outcome too much and then you let some things stay. Desserts are supposed to contain some sugar or other sweetener. Scrambled eggs and omelets may taste better with a little bit of cheese. Vegetables sautéed or roasted in oil taste richer. Bread is delicious with a little bit of butter or olive oil. Meals with no fat or sugar are dull and unsatisfying, so let yourself live a little. You don't have to go overboard.

I learned this lesson the hard way when I was first developing some of my BethennyBakes products and I tried making them completely fat-free. Trust me, you don't get extra points for fat-free. No one cares. The taste isn't as good. If you are going to eat, it should taste fantastic. A fat-free muffin, cookie, or cupcake does not taste fantastic, so why bother? Sorry, no extra credit for fat-free.

When I used to have a lot of food noise, I was terrified of fat, but now I've learned that if you cut out every single thing you think might have too many calories or too much fat, nobody (including you) is going to like the taste. Taste should be your first priority. Then work on making it better for you. If something doesn't give in your recipes, then you'll end up overeating because you feel too deprived.

Rule 4: Embrace the "It Ain't Worth It" Moment

Sometimes when I'm developing a recipe, I'm trying to do all the right things, but at some point when something isn't working or I can't find the right ingredient, it just gets too hard. That's when I embrace the "It Ain't Worth It" moment.

If you tear your stocking on the run, you might have to go out and buy a new pair because you don't have time to go home and figure out an alternative. If your shoes really hurt and you've got to walk, you may have to just go with the comfortable ones. No time to get to the salon or your flat-iron session isn't working out? Sometimes it's just easier to wear a hat or a ponytail or go with the curly look.

When I was testing the Lighter Chicken Pot Pie for this cookbook, I wanted to use an organic whole-wheat piecrust, but I couldn't find any premade whole-wheat piecrusts that would work for a double-crust pie. I could only find the easy folded refrigerated crust. I was not going to make a crust from scratch (see Rule 1), but the premade crust contained white flour and some lard. I thought about using the lard crust over the top of the frozen whole-wheat crust and then I realized: Who is going to bother to do that? So the easy crust has some lard in it. That makes it flakier, and as you know from Rule 3, something's got to give. The filling of the pie is low-fat, so the crust was what had to give in this situation. The amount of crust you will eat in one serving of my Lighter Chicken Pot Pie is maybe 120 calories. Better yet, just eat half the crust. The crust you will eat is not a big deal, so don't worry about it. Look for whole wheat, and if you can't find it, move on. It's just not worth the stress.

Rule 5: Taste As You Go

Good cooks always taste their food as they cook it. Amateur cooks just mix it all up and cross their fingers that it will taste okay when it's all done. Just as you look in the mirror before you go out for a special occasion, you should never serve food without tasting it first. I'm not talking about tasting a whole meal's worth of calories before the food gets to the table. I'm talking about taking tiny bites and sips along the way.

Tasting is an important way to learn what a recipe needs and to discover how flavors change as they cook longer. As you taste, keep gauging whether something needs a little more salt or pepper or lemon juice or spice. Add just a little at a time because you can always add more, but you can't always make something less salty or less spicy (although see Chapter 5 for some tips on fixing seasoning mistakes).

Rule 6: *Mise en Place*— the French Cooking Term You *Should* Know

I'm not one of those chefs who likes to throw French words around. I don't think many of them are very useful to people cooking dinner at home. This term, however, is an exception. *Mise en place*, pronounced meez-ahn-plahs (barely pronounce the *n*), means "put in place."

This is like laying out your clothes the night before so that you have everything you need to get ready in the morning. In cooking, it means that you get all your tools and all your ingredients ready before you turn on a burner or grease a single pan. This is why cooking looks so easy on cooking shows. Everything is prepared, measured, and set out beforehand. You can do this at home. Chop and measure all the vegetables. Be sure the meat is defrosted. Premeasure the flour, sugar, baking powder, and cinnamon. Put all the ingredients out. I like to put everything in small ramekins or small glass bowls. Will you need a sifter? A citrus juicer? A whisk? Pull them out before you start.

Mise en place requires reading the whole recipe before you start. This is so important! I cannot tell you how many times I have completely screwed up a recipe by not reading the whole thing first. If you are just beginning to get comfortable in the kitchen (or even if you are already experienced but want to follow a recipe), reading the recipe first, then assembling your ingredients and tools, will make cooking a hundred times easier. There won't be any surprises. Read the whole recipe so that you can conceptualize it and be thinking about it before you start cooking. Cooking will become practically effortless when you get in the habit of *mise en place*.

However, in the spirit of full disclosure, I will admit to you that as much as I think it's a good idea, I don't always do *mise en place*. It really does help and I'm always glad when I do it. In a perfect world, I would always do this, but my world isn't perfect and neither is yours. I'm especially likely to do this if someone is helping me, but sometimes I don't and sometimes I mess up. That's life. Just do your best.

Rule 7: Memorize a Few Basics

I'll get into some more detailed chef techniques in Chapter 6 that will give you superior results and make cooking easier. First, though, it will be very helpful to memorize a few key basics that you will need to know again and again.

If you memorize these, you won't have to keep running to your computer to Google the answers, like how many tablespoons in a cup or whether you can bake those muffins without using eggs. You might already know some of these basics. If you commit all of them to memory right now (or do one a day until you know them all), you'll be forever glad you did. This information is particularly helpful when you want to double a recipe or cut it in half, or when you are out of something and you want to feel more confident that something else will work in its place:

- 3 teaspoons = 1 tablespoon
- 4 tablespoons = ¼ cup
- 16 tablespoons = 1 cup
- 2 tablespoons = 1 fluid ounce
- 8 fluid ounces = 1 cup
- 2 cups = 16 ounces = 1 pint
- 2 pints = 4 cups = 1 quart
- 4 quarts = 16 cups = 1 gallon
- 1 tablespoon chopped fresh herbs = 1 teaspoon crumbled dried herbs
- Measure carefully when baking. Don't worry so much about it for other kinds of cooking.
- Whenever a recipe refers to an egg, in any cookbook anywhere, it means a large egg. But I've never really noticed egg size and this has never once ruined any of my recipes.

For Vegetarians and Vegans

- You can almost always use extra-firm tofu instead of any meat, poultry, or fish, in an equivalent weight. You can almost always prepare it exactly the same way—marinated, seasoned, grilled, fried, baked, sautéed, and so on. It will soak up the flavors of the other ingredients better and have a meatier texture if it is well drained before marinating or cooking. Open and drain the water, then blot the tofu with paper towels. For even better drainage, wrap it in more paper towels and weigh it down with a cutting board for about ten minutes.

- If you want to leave eggs out of your baking, you can buy egg replacement powder (made by Ener-G; this is a popular ingredient in vegan cooking) or substitute about ¼ cup of mashed banana, plain yogurt, or applesauce per egg. Experiment to see what works in any given recipe. This doesn't always work, so experiment with care.
- 1 cup milk can be any milk: cow, soy, rice, almond, and so forth.
- 1 cup yogurt can be low-fat Fage brand or other Greek yogurt, or soy yogurt.
- You can always substitute soy or rice cheese for regular cheese. Follow Your Heart Vegan Gourmet is a good brand that doesn't contain any casein, a milk product in many of the so-called nondairy cheeses. It comes in a variety of flavors. Nondairy cheese is very processed, but I still use it because I don't like to eat a lot of dairy. Find what you like and what you are willing to try.

Rule 8: Presentation Is Everything

It doesn't matter how expensive your shoes are or what designer made your dress if you wear it wrinkled or dirty or you look sloppy or mismatched. Food can taste good, but if it doesn't look good and it isn't presented nicely, people (including you, the cook) won't necessarily enjoy it. You eat with your eyes first, so how food looks really does matter. This is where it's worth taking extra time to make your food really special. Think about the food you would get at a spa or at a nice restaurant. These places know how to make food look delicious by using a lot of contrasting natural colors and textures, like fresh lemon zest over fish and fresh parsley over salsa. Take the time to do this. Making meals into events makes food feel and taste more special. You'll be more likely to savor it and eat less because it will be more satisfying.

Presentation means two things: (1) Arrange food nicely. Garnish your dishes with bright, fresh raw vegetables, fruit, or herb sprigs. Contrast colors in your salads and between main and side dishes. Remember that naturally colorful foods are better for you. (2) Especially when entertaining, serve food creatively. Use platters, stack plates on bowls, drape fabric around a buffet, put fresh flowers on the table, light candles, and buy inexpensive themed serving pieces, especially for entertaining (see Chapter 14 for some party-specific serving ideas). Even if you're dining alone, use your nice dishes, light a candle, and design your plate artfully. Make your meal into an event. Enjoy your food, appreciating not only how it tastes but also how it looks. You'll get a lot more out of the experience, you'll eat more slowly, and you'll probably digest your food better.

Rule 9: Utilize the Leftovers

Remember those plastic containers I suggested you include as part of your kitchen inventory in Chapter 2? This is where you use them. Label the containers and put leftovers into meal-size portions. Every time you put one of these clearly labeled meals in the freezer, that's one more day in the future that you won't have to cook.

This is also a better approach than storing multiple servings in large containers. Looking into a messy bag of leftovers isn't very appealing, but individual portions nicely arranged in small containers make it easy for anybody in the family to enjoy one serving of that meal again at their convenience. These plastic containers are also great for storing leftovers you bring home from a restaurant or for saving food from a big meal. For example, after Thanksgiving, store turkey, butternut squash puree, and green bean casserole in separate serving-size containers. Take them out, warm them up, and you have a three-course meal. For more ideas on creative ways to use leftovers, see Chapter 4.

Rule 10: Minimize Cleanup

Do you have a husband who says, "Honey, you did all that work to make dinner and I appreciate it so much. Go relax, my darling. Put your feet up. I'll clean the kitchen, love of my life"? And then you woke up. Or, maybe you're in the first six months of your relationship and you're still having sex every day. Okay, I know that some husbands are very helpful and some are even neat freaks, but if your husband is more like the guy who will put away one dish before realizing the game is on, this rule is for you.

Seriously, how annoying is cleanup? It's the worst part of cooking. Many people who say they hate to cook really mean they hate to clean up afterward. Cooking is easy. Cleaning up is hard. Since you can't take all your dishes, pots, and pans to the dry cleaner, why should you have to suffer alone? There are great ways to make cleanup easier if you are cooking for yourself, but if anybody else is benefitting from your new culinary skills, they need to understand that there is a price.

I hate cleanup. It gives me anxiety. Whenever my weekly housekeeper comes and cleans my kitchen, I vow to never cook again and never to mess up my perfect kitchen. I treat my kitchen like it's a brand-new car and can't be touched by human hands. Then reality sets in. If you are going to cook, somebody has to clean, and cleaning isn't so bad if you share the burden. Tell your husband you'll give him a little extra love in the bedroom for some help in the kitchen. Assign specific chores to people so that nobody gets away without helping: "You clear the table, you clean the salad dishes, you rinse, and I'll load the dishwasher." Tell your girlfriends, your kids, and your relatives that if they do even 25 percent of the cleanup, you will cook for them anytime, anywhere. Every little bit helps, and once somebody starts pitching in to help, they will usually do at least half the work.

Don't be afraid to resort to bribery to get people to help you. Make the favorite foods of each member of your family, then designate cleanup helpers. They'll be so satisfied that they shouldn't mind at all. Bribery is perfectly acceptable if used for good, not evil—and cleaning your kitchen is always good.

But even half the work can be daunting, so I'm giving you a helping hand already. None of the recipes in this book will involve heavy cleanup. Part of the Skinnygirl philosophy of cooking is to keep it light and easy so that cleanup will always be minimal. The goal is to get you back into the kitchen, not to panic you so that you never want to go in there again. Here are some more things to try:

- Think about the whole meal as you cook. If a meal has a roasted meat and a sautéed vegetable, sauté the vegetable in an ovenproof pan, set the vegetable aside, and roast the meat in that same pan. You've already got the flavors of roasted vegetables, which will complement the meat.
- If you are tossing a salad in a simple vinaigrette, whisk the vinaigrette in the bottom of the salad bowl before you put in the vegetables. Then add your greens and toss everything together. One bowl, minimal mess.
- If you need to mix turkey burgers, look at the turkey meat container. Is it one of those fairly deep plastic trays? Can you mix the turkey meat right in there without messing up a bowl? Then you can just throw that container away or recycle it. You would be throwing it away, anyway.
- Instead of messing up your counters or cutting boards, use butcher paper to hold seasoned meat or sliced vegetables before you put them on the grill.
- I put butcher paper, foil, or parchment paper on cutting boards, baking sheets, roasting pans, and serving platters to minimize cleanup. It took me ten years to figure out that doing this simple thing could save me so much effort!
- Use jars or bottles of oil or vinegar that are almost empty to mix, serve, and store dressing.
- When pulling out big pieces of equipment like a food processor, do as many things as you can with it so that you only have to clean it once. Start with simpler ingredients and later do the ones with more fragrant flavors. Chop broccoli and then rinse, then grate Parmesan and rinse, then do garlic and onions last so that their strong flavors don't transfer to other foods. Honestly though, I almost never use my food processor, except when preparing large quantities of food for, say, Thanksgiving. I'd rather do most of

those jobs with my chef's knife and a cutting board or with my immersion blender.

- Presentation is important, but you still don't need to mess up more plates and platters than necessary. Decide if you're plating your family's or guests' food. If so, then go from pan to plate. The platter is just an unnecessary middle step. Put the cooking pan on a trivet and it can be its own serving platter. Unless this is a fancy dinner (most aren't really), you don't need separate salad plates, bread plates, and so on. Put everything on one plate (with the exception of the soup).

Actually, I'm so committed to this last concept that I'm considering pulling up a stool in front of the stove and eating right out of the pan. (Because of *Naturally Thin*, you already know you should never eat standing up.) I wonder how many stools I could fit in front of my stove . . . this could be my next dinner party.

There you have it: ten rules for the Skinnygirl chef. Learn them, live them, and love cooking.

Chapter 4

Use What You Have: Core Concepts

I say it again and again throughout this book, in the rules, in the recipes, and whenever it's relevant, because this is one of the most important things I want you to understand about cooking for yourself at home: *Use what you have!*

The majority of the recipes I invent or renovate are born this way. Obviously, you will need to go to the store and buy food, but it's so easy to overspend when you don't consider what you already have. You'll save money, you'll be "greener," and you'll be less wasteful if you learn how to cook with what you actually have and use those ingredients in what you are making.

The whole point of Chapter 2—giving you a refrigerator and a pantry list of "classics" and "accessories"—is for you to actually have things to use. You can make a good meal or a snack without ever having to go out and buy anything. Keep your kitchen stocked with the items on those lists and you're good to go.

Recipes aren't absolutes. They are guides. I really want you to get to the point where you are thinking for yourself in the kitchen and coming up with your own ideas about how to use what you have. I want you to think: I want a salad. What do I have that will make it interesting? Then I want you to be able to look into your refrigerator and pantry and get inspired: Pine nuts and Parmesan! Walnuts and dried cranberries! How about a dressing made up of this leftover pesto? What about these leftover roasted vegetables?

Let's say you want to make one of the recipes from this book. Maybe you are having a party and you want to serve the artichoke and spinach dip. How do you use what you have? Let's do a tutorial. Let's look at that ingredients list (which you can also find on page 239, along with the full recipe) to see what substitutions you can use and when substituting doesn't really work, so you can start to think outside the recipe.

Guilt-Free Artichoke and Spinach Dip

1 package (about 9 ounces) frozen artichokes, defrosted and drained

What if you can't find frozen artichokes in your grocery store? Are you forbidden from ever enjoying the recipe? Of course not. If you can only find canned artichoke hearts, drain them well and use those. If you can only find the little jars of marinated ones, rinse them well and use those. If worst comes to worst, just use twice the amount of spinach and forget the artichokes.

1 package (about 9 ounces) frozen spinach, defrosted and drained

I can't imagine a grocery store without frozen spinach, but if you are out and haven't restocked yet, and you happen to have a bag of fresh spinach, finely chop the spinach and heat it with a little water in a covered pan until it cooks down and looks like defrosted frozen spinach. As for canned spinach, that's where I draw the line, because it's disgusting.

¼ cup freshly grated Parmesan cheese, divided (grate it yourself)

The Parmesan in the can that is pre-grated doesn't taste anything like freshly grated Parmesan, so this is another item that you should always stock. But what if you don't have any? If you have Romano cheese, use that. You could also use Pecorino (a sheep's milk cheese) or even feta or goat cheese. Or, just replace the Parmesan with double the amount of any other shredded cheese. It won't have that classic Parmesan "bite," but it will still be creamy and cheesy and good. Drawing the line at the canned Parmesan cheese is where it matters—but if all you have is the can? Use it, taste it, fix it. You can compensate in other ways with fresh herbs. Just keep tasting and adjusting until you like how it tastes.

¼ cup shredded Monterey Jack cheese

If you don't have Monterey Jack cheese but you do have mozzarella, you could use that, but the results will taste a little different. You could also substitute white cheddar or another white cheese like Edam or even smoked Gouda, for a different taste. If you only have shredded Colby-Jack, you could use that. There is no science to this. The recipe calls for Monterey Jack because that's what *I* happened to have when I made this.

¼ cup part-skim ricotta cheese

If you are out of ricotta, substitute low-fat cottage cheese whipped in the blender for a few seconds to smooth out the curd, or silken tofu with a sprinkle of salt, which will both give similar results to the ricotta.

8 ounces reduced-fat or soy cream cheese (like Tofutti)

If you don't have low-fat cream cheese but you do have low-fat sour cream, Greek yogurt, or plain soy yogurt, you could substitute those. Yogurt will make the dip creamier and less cheesy, but it will still be good.

2 tablespoons nondairy or low-fat mayonnaise

You should always have some kind of mayonnaise in your refrigerator. Use any kind you have. Low-fat and nondairy versions are preferable.

½ tablespoon lemon juice

You should always have fresh lemons in your refrigerator, but if you don't, you could use bottled lemon juice in this recipe because it doesn't require very much. Or, go for a more exotic taste and use lime juice, if that's what you have.

1 clove garlic, minced

If you don't have fresh garlic, you could use jarred minced garlic. The amount is small, so it won't really affect the taste. One-half teaspoon minced garlic equals one clove. You could also use ½ teaspoon garlic powder.

¾ teaspoon salt and *½ teaspoon black pepper*

Garlic salt, sea salt, kosher salt—you have some kind of salt, right? Black pepper could be white pepper, although, personally, I am not a fan of white pepper.

2 dashes Tabasco sauce

If you don't have Tabasco, use any other hot sauce, or a dash of cayenne pepper, or ½ teaspoon red pepper flakes.

Using what you have is even easier to illustrate when you are talking about foods like salads, soups, and casseroles, but I understand it can be difficult to know what you can use in place of what ingredient. That's why I created the Use-What-You-Have Substitution List.

Use-What-You-Have Substitution List

I made this list so that you could start teaching yourself to break free from recipes by using what you have instead of following a recipe to the letter. This list will help you understand, when you are in your kitchen with a recipe in front of you, exactly what you can do to substitute for a missing ingredient. Use this list with creativity, but also with caution. Substituting ingredients *will change the result*. To maximize your success, read this list through so you understand what kinds of substitutions *usually* work, and what kinds of substitutions are riskier. Remember to *pay attention* to the results to figure out what you like, what works, and what you probably won't try again. I never used to write anything down, but now I do so I remember what worked. You can do that, too.

You can usually substitute any ingredient in each category, but note exceptions:

Vegetables and Fruits

Any root vegetable: carrots, parsnips, turnips, beets, or any potatoes.

Any potato: russet, white, Yukon gold, red, sweet potatoes/ yams, or even any winter squash. Sometimes you can substitute potatoes for root vegetables, and vice versa.

Any onion in the onion family: white, yellow, or red onions, leeks, shallots, scallions, and even chives when the recipe calls for a small amount or a garnish.

Any leafy lettuce: romaine, red lettuce, butter lettuce, mixed baby greens, baby spinach, arugula, even finely shredded cabbage, especially Napa or Savoy.

Any cooking greens: kale, Swiss chard, collard greens, mustard greens, beet greens, and so on. Each tastes slightly different, so be aware of that. Raw foodists eat greens like kale and collards without cooking them.

Any garden vegetable: zucchini, bell peppers, broccoli, cauliflower, green beans, brussels sprouts, asparagus, eggplant, summer squash, cabbage, bok choy, soy beans, and so on. When roasting, cooking time will be longer for firmer vegetables and shorter for softer ones.

Any winter squash: butternut, acorn, pumpkin, or spaghetti squash, or substitute sweet potatoes or yams. Sometimes these can stand in for potatoes or root vegetables.

Any peas or beans: black beans, pinto beans, white beans, navy beans, red beans, soy beans, chickpeas, lentils, black-eyed peas, lima beans, or green peas.

Fresh tomatoes or canned tomatoes when cooked (use only fresh
when they need to be raw).

Any orchard fruit: apples, pears, peaches, nectarines, or plums.

Any berry: strawberries, blackberries, raspberries, or blueberries.

HERB BLURB

Fresh herbs and dried herbs are not necessarily interchangeable. Dried herbs have a more intense taste so you need less, and in some recipes that call for fresh herbs, dried just won't taste very good. You can understand the difference if you consider the difference between a fresh Pomodoro sauce, which is fresh tomatoes chopped with fresh basil, and an old-school marinara with its deep, rich flavors from slow cooking. Fresh herbs make sense in the Pomodoro; dried herbs make sense in the marinara.

If it really doesn't matter whether you use fresh or dried herbs, I'll indicate that in the Use-What-You-Have Variations list after a recipe, but in general, I'll direct you to substitute fresh green leafy herbs (like parsley or basil) for other fresh leafy herbs (like cilantro or dill), and dried herbs (like oregano or sage) for other dried herbs (like thyme or tarragon).

Grains, Nuts, and Seeds

Any grain: rice (preferably brown), quinoa, spelt, bulgur (the
grain in tabbouleh), pasta (any shape, preferably whole grain),
oats, barley, millet, whole-grain cornmeal, couscous, or Israeli
couscous. Different grains require different cooking times, so if
you do substitute one grain for another, check the directions on
the package.

Any flour: oat, whole-wheat pastry, whole wheat, brown rice
(different flours will impact the flavor and texture of baked
goods, sometimes a lot).

Any nut: walnuts, slivered or sliced almonds, pine nuts, pecans, cashews, and so on.

Any nut butters: peanut, almond, cashew, sesame.

Any seed: sunflower, pumpkin, sesame, and so on. Sometimes you can substitute seeds for nuts.

Dairy

Any hard, highly flavored grating cheese: Parmesan, Romano, or Pecorino.

Any medium-soft cheese: cheddar, Monterey Jack, Colby, Gouda, Edam, mozzarella, farmer's cheese, or nondairy cheese.

Any soft cheese: feta, chèvre, or goat cheese, or even silken tofu with a sprinkle of salt.

Any fermented dairy product: plain yogurt, Greek yogurt, soy yogurt, low-fat sour cream, vegan sour cream, or buttermilk.

Any cream cheese: low-fat cream cheese, regular cream cheese, Neufchâtel, nondairy cream cheese, mascarpone, or ricotta.

Any salt, any black pepper.

Any milk: cow, soy, rice, almond, coconut, hazelnut, or hemp.

Oils, Vinegars, and Citrus

Any oil or melted fat: canola, vegetable, olive, coconut, butter, non-dairy butter. *However,* if you are using the oil in a salad dressing or in any other form where it is not cooked, use high-quality cold-pressed oil, such as extra-virgin olive oil, flavored oils like herb oils, fancy nut oils, or truffle oil. When you are *cooking* with an oil, use any cooking oil, such as canola oil, regular olive oil, vegetable oil, corn oil, and so on.

Any vinegar: white, apple cider, champagne, rice, wine, or herb-infused.

Any citrus juice: lemon, lime, orange, grapefruit. However, consider first if you think the flavor will work.

Baking

Eggs: 1 egg for 2 egg whites or vice versa. Or, if you want to avoid eggs (for you vegans), substitute any of the following in baking for 1 egg: ½ banana, ½ cup pumpkin puree (not pumpkin pie mix), ½ cup butternut squash puree, ½ cup pureed fruit, ½ cup any fruit baby food, or egg substitute powder (like Ener-G).

Any dry sweetener: raw sugar, Sucanat, or Florida Crystals (turbinado).

Any liquid sweetener: honey, maple syrup, agave nectar, brown rice syrup, or molasses (use less molasses—it's very strong). Usually, substitute granulated sweeteners for each other only, and liquid sweeteners for each other only, unless a recipe indicates they are interchangeable.

(By the way, I do *not* generally recommend using any artificial sweeteners, although I do sometimes put a packet of Splenda in my coffee.)

SHOULD YOU USE STEVIA?

Some people love to use Stevia as a sweetener instead of sugar. Personally, I don't use it. Stevia is a naturally sweet herb sold in health food stores, but using it can be tricky. It doesn't taste good in everything. It's like turning twenty-one and taking your first shot of tequila—you might not realize how strong it is. Me, I can do three shots of tequila without a problem, but I still can't figure out how to use Stevia the right way, so try it if you want to, but just be careful and err on the side of less.

Any extracts: vanilla, almond, orange, raspberry, maple, coconut, banana, and so on. There are so many different kinds of extracts to try, so be creative but also think about what you are making. What kind of extract would work best for the flavors of your dish?

Cocktails

Any clear liquor for any other clear liquor: tequila, vodka, rum, or gin. You can also change out citrus juices (lime for lemon or orange), and you can swap out flavored citrus liqueurs, such as Grand Marnier for Cointreau for Triple Sec, and for nut liqueurs such as amaretto for Frangelico or macadamia nut liqueur.

Chapter 5

Learn from My Kitchen Blunders

*J*ust because I'm a chef and went to cooking school does not mean that everything I attempt in the kitchen comes out totally delicious and perfect. In fact, sometimes it's the exact opposite. Making mistakes in the kitchen is a little like thinking you look really great in an outfit, then ending up on the worst-dressed list. The more you understand and practice cooking, the better you will get at avoiding blunders.

I learned a lot in cooking school, but I've learned a lot more since then by figuring out what works and what doesn't. I use what I have, and when the result really matters, I rely on things that I know work. Otherwise, I like to take risks, try things, and see what happens. Sometimes the results are great. I find a new favorite recipe. Sometimes . . . well, let's just say I've had my fair share of blunders.

Anybody can cook, but anybody can mess up, too. The other day, I was working on a healthy pancake recipe and the result was just a mess. The pancakes were really horrible. My fiancé, Jason, laughed at me and said, "You're a chef and you can't make pancakes?" I have attempted healthful versions of cookies that ran together all over the baking sheet because of ingredient substitutions that didn't work.

As I was working on recipes for this book, I tried to make a low-fat key lime pie. That did *not* work. It wouldn't set. It just stayed completely liquid, and I totally messed up my kitchen and then I had to toss it. You'll notice there is no recipe in this book for low-fat key lime pie. I'll figure out a way to make it work, but it just wasn't going to happen this time. Then there was the time I tried to use avocado as the main fat in a pan of brownies. I've heard of people doing this and saying it's a great idea, but I got green mushy brownies. Yuck.

Making mistakes can be so frustrating. I have wanted to move out of my apartment after having to dump an entire pan of brownies into the garbage, melting the garbage bag. I've looked into the oven to see that my carrot cake muffins boiled over and exploded because I used too much liquid sweetener. They dripped down through the grates and spread all over the bottom of the oven. Do I have to explain what it's like to clean burnt sugar batter off the oven floor? Now I know to keep a sheet of foil or an oven liner in the bottom of my oven. If only I would have thought of that before those fateful carrot cake muffins. Seriously, I almost lost it, I was about to cry, trying to scrape the hardened batter, and at one point, my assistant had to tell me to just step away and get out of the kitchen. She went in there with a level head and cleaned it up.

I don't want you to think that if you make a mistake in the kitchen and something doesn't turn out the way you planned—or is just plain horrible—that you are a bad cook or that you can't cook. As long as you are paying attention and learning from your mistakes, you'll keep getting better and better. You just have to have a sense of humor about it. You don't have to take cooking that seriously. Sometimes you will. Sometimes you will be horribly disappointed. And sometimes, much more often than not, when everything works, you'll see why being adventurous in cooking is worth it. Besides, kitchen disasters make for great stories and lessons learned. How else would I write this chapter?

Remember as you cook, especially in the middle of a cooking disaster, this rule: "Don't be a hero." The only thing smart about my key lime pie attempt was the graham cracker crust that I bought at the store. Keep things simple so that when a recipe doesn't work or isn't all that great, you won't have invested too much of your time in vain. If I would have bothered to make a homemade crust and then had to throw it all away, I would have been even more frustrated! Cut your losses. Buy the premade graham cracker crust if you are experimenting. Then when you know the recipe works, you can invest more time in the other details, like a homemade crust.

Also, remember from *Naturally Thin* that if you don't really like something, *you don't have to eat it*. Better to throw it away and "waste" it than put it in your body for no good reason. It's a bigger waste to eat food you don't really love.

This chapter isn't meant to discourage you. Most of the time, your creations are going to be great. I just want to remind you that even the most experienced cooks screw up sometimes. These stories are meant to amuse you and to be a kind of commiseration when your recipe doesn't work, either.

My "Oops" Moments

One of the reasons I always advise getting cookware that can go into the oven is because I once made a frittata and put it in the oven to finish it.

It was beautiful, but when I put it in the oven, the oven melted the handle right off the pan. I didn't realize this until I tried to take it out of the oven and the whole thing fell on the floor because the handle broke off. I'm going to admit this—I picked it up off the floor and served it. Thank God this didn't happen when cooking for a client! When my assistant, Julie, reads this, she is going to pee her pants because she was one of the people who was there that night. I told them that the earthy taste was the mushrooms. Anyway, those were the same friends who taught me about the three-second rule.

I dropped a turkey on the floor once, too. I picked it up, rinsed it off, put it back into the oven, then served it. Maybe this is why I don't have my own restaurant. I'd be sued. I'm certainly not recommending that you serve food that you dropped on the floor. However, I am just saying that it's easy to get distracted and be doing too many things at once and not realize that you don't have a firm grip on something and suddenly you've lost control of it and it's on the floor.

These disasters could have been worse. I have a friend whose mother dropped a hot fruit pie on her foot and ended up in the emergency room with third-degree burns. I have a scar on my arm from burning myself on a bagel. In fact, most chefs have a lot of scars on their hands and arms from working in crowded restaurant kitchens, so a few scars can give you cooking clout. Not that they are necessary to be a good cook, of course, but we all have clumsy moments. The lesson is that whenever you are taking something out of the oven or moving it from the stove to the oven, you have to be very careful. Pay attention to what you are doing and you'll be a lot less likely to drop your carefully prepared dinner on the floor. Also, never use a wet towel to take anything hot off the stove or out of the oven. People think using a wet towel is fine, but heat travels right through water and will burn your hand.

Other "oops" moments have involved mistaken ingredients. My best one while writing this cookbook was when I was working on the recipe for a low-fat pasta carbonara. You might remember on the second season of *The Real Housewives* when I made Pasta Carbonara (page 147), which normally is the last thing I would make because it's one of the most high-fat dishes on the planet—made with butter, bacon, and cheese. Of course, that inspired me to create a lower-fat version, but when I made the one for this book, I accidentally used vanilla soy milk instead of plain soy milk! It was not good. Not good at all. Imagine a vanilla latte with bacon. Yeah. What a disaster. My fiancé is so sweet that he ate it, even though it was vile. I called it Café Latte Carbonara. If I would have been paying closer attention to what I was doing, I wouldn't have used vanilla soy milk. Obviously.

Of course, as I mentioned in a previous chapter, sometimes a mistake can turn into a happy accident. That same day, I accidentally used the vanilla soy milk instead of regular soy milk while testing my Ricotta Cheesecake recipe (page 195). The results were fantastic, and vanilla soy milk became an integral part of the recipe. This is why you shouldn't be afraid to make mistakes. Sometimes you'll love the results. Roses have petals and thorns, and my low-fat cheesecake was the petal. The Café Latte Carbonara was the thorn.

When I first tried to lighten up Green Bean Casserole (page 220), I forgot to drain the green beans after cooking them in chicken broth. I added the rest of the ingredients and the result was a soupy mess—green bean casserole soup. I had to drain the whole thing, losing most of the mushroom soup. What a waste. When I added the cream cheese, the result was actually really good, but I've since revised this recipe so that you aren't wasting anything.

My Red Velvet Cake (page 186) did not turn out red at all. I had the idea of using nutritious beet juice instead of food coloring, as you would use in traditional red velvet cake. The batter was a beautiful bright pink, so I thought I was on the right track, but after it baked, it didn't look red at all, or even pink. It was also a very delicate cake, and when one of my testers made it, the cake completely fell apart when she tried to take it out of the pan. She didn't use the parchment paper because she thought her nonstick pans would be good enough. They weren't. However, instead of throwing it all away, she broke it into pieces, layered it with pudding and strawberries in a glass bowl, and topped it with the frosting. Her kids devoured the "Red Velvet Trifle" (even though it wasn't red), which she made by using what she had to fix her disaster. As I'm writing this, I am thinking that mashed beets would have been an even better addition. I'll try that next time.

A good way to make delicate cake recipes is to use a release pan (sometimes called a springform pan) so that you don't have to turn it out of the pan and risk breaking it. I also like to make cupcakes using liners—the easiest option of all.

Most kitchen disasters happen because (1) you aren't paying attention, (2) you are going too fast, (3) you didn't follow the instructions, or (4) you were taking a risk, trying something new. I keep telling you *not* to be chained to a recipe's instructions, but when you do deviate, you have to realize that it might work or it might not. The more you cook, the more you get a sense for when your deviations will work and when they won't, but even the most experienced cook will sometimes make a wrong decision.

The best way to minimize kitchen disasters is to pay attention to what you are doing so you don't have a klutzy moment and you don't accidentally put vanilla soy milk into your pasta. However, I'll never tell you not to try something new or take a risk. That's part of the fun and creativity of cooking.

Your Fix-It Guide

The basic tastes that season or flavor foods are salt, sugar, and acid. Fat also adds flavor. When you have all these flavoring agents, you can learn how to season any food and to correct an overseasoned dish. The key is to balance these flavors. When a food is too salty, try adding a little more sugar (raw sugar, honey, agave syrup, molasses, maple syrup) and acid (lemon juice, lime juice, vinegar). When a food is too sweet, try adding more salt and acid. When a food is too acidic, try adding more sugar and salt. Each one of these three elements can be balanced using the other two. It's like magic.

When a food is too anything, diluting it can also be a lifesaver. Add more of the other ingredients—water, flour, milk, or broth. Of course, sometimes an overseasoned dish can't be saved. If you accidentally dumped a whole salt shaker into your soup or way too many chili peppers into your chili, it might be inedible. You can try to fix your dish, but at some point you have to stop chasing it. I made soup once and put in too much apple cider vinegar. I kept trying to adjust and fix it, but it kept getting away from me and finally I had to give up. It wasn't worth fixing because it was never going to be good.

If you burn a dish, you will also have to toss it. Don't just serve the unburned part, because the entire dish will have the burned flavor. The most important key to seasoning is always to season in small increments and taste constantly so that you can monitor how the flavors in your food are developing. A little salt, taste, a little more salt, taste, a little lemon juice, taste, a little sugar, taste. As you cook something, the flavors change. Water evaporates and spice or salt gets stronger. Flavors blend together. Food also tastes different at different temperatures, so flavors you couldn't taste when a dish is steaming hot might be much more obvious as the dish cools down. That's why it's so important to taste as you go.

Another important thing to remember is to save some of your seasoning for the end. Make a final seasoning adjustment just before serving. You want to know exactly how that dish will taste on the plate.

Here are some other things you can do when your flavors are out of whack:

• If your food is too bland: This is the best problem you can possibly have. Bland food just needs more salt, sugar, acid, or spice. Sometimes it just needs that ineffable quality I call "zip." That might come from pepper or spices, seasoning mixes, or the freshness of herbs. In general, people tend to be stingy with salt because they think it is bad for them. Processed foods have tons of salt, but if you are making your own food from scratch, you don't have to worry about using salt in amounts that will flavor the food. Almost all food can benefit from a little bit of salt, which brings out food's natural flavor. Then think about what else might give the dish character: Black and red pepper add spice. Acid, like a squeeze of fresh lemon or lime juice or a splash of vinegar, will add brightness and tang. Sugar adds sweetness, of course, and a chopped fresh herb or a sprinkle of ground spice can also bring a bland dish alive again. I also like to add Worcestershire sauce for "zip."

The key here is to *taste as you go* and add just a little bit of seasoning at a time until you like the flavor.

- If your food is too salty: You might have heard that you can add a raw potato to your overly salty soup and it will absorb the salt. Some sources say that's actually an old wives' tale and it doesn't work, while other people swear by it. I don't know if it works because I've never tried it, but if you really went overboard with the salt and you have a potato lying around, it couldn't hurt. However, the best way to avoid this very common mistake is to always salt on the cautious side and keep tasting as you go, adding just a little bit at a time so that you know when the soup tastes perfect.

Also remember the sacred trio of salt, sugar, and acid. If you accidentally pour in too much salt, a little bit of sweetener, like raw sugar or honey, and a little bit of acid, like fresh lemon juice, can balance out the saltiness.

You might also need to add more water to dilute the salt. A few more chopped vegetables might help, too. Remember to cut your losses if you've ruined the dish. You have to know when to hold 'em and know when to fold 'em.

If your salad dressing is too salty, add a little more oil (to dilute), citrus or vinegar (acid), and sugar or honey. Water can help, too.

- If your food is too sour: Add a little more sweetener and salt to balance too much acid. Also, add more liquid to dilute the sour flavor.

- If your food is too sweet: A little salt and some acid will cut the cloying sweetness. More liquid can, too, although don't add liquid out of proportion in a baking recipe or you could ruin the result.

- If your food is too spicy: If you've added too many hot peppers to your chili or salsa, or too many red pepper flakes to your casserole, you can reduce the effect by diluting it with more liquid or chopped vegetables (like juicy tomatoes).

Creamy foods have a cooling effect and can reduce the impact of hot pepper spice when they are appropriate for the dish. Just before serving, stir in a little bit of yogurt, sour cream, or milk, or top the food with some yogurt or sour cream and a little cheese.

Again, however, the best way to avoid this mistake is to add seasonings, including hot spices, a little at a time and taste as you go. Remember that food concentrates as it cooks and more water evaporates, so something that is a little bit spicy (or salty) at first will get spicier (or saltier) the longer you cook it.

Also remember to leave some spice for the end. Salt and spices can intensify while you are cooking. When I was working on the Boyfriend Roast Chicken recipe (page 130), I salted the chicken and put it on top of the vegetables and onions. The salt melted off the skin and dripped down all over the vegetables underneath the chicken, so they turned out too salty. Salting the chicken more lightly and not salting the vegetables, then adding more salt at the end, made all the difference.

I want to leave you with the thought that you *will* make mistakes, as do I, and *that's okay*. That's how we learn and take it to the next level, so relax, accept that mistakes will happen, don't be afraid to take chances, and always be ready to *use what you have* to try to fix what went wrong. And when it doesn't work? Just throw it away and start over . . . or call the bakery.

Chapter 6

Channeling Your Inner Chef

*C*ooking can be easy, but knowing a few chef's tricks will definitely make it easier. In this chapter, I'm going to share those secrets with you so that you don't have to go to cooking school to feel like a chef.

In order to channel your inner chef, you have to start thinking like a chef. Taste is the first priority, not blind adherence to a recipe. Chefs don't rely on recipes. They often consult recipes for inspiration or research, but they use those concepts and take them in their own direction. You can do that, too, especially if you start seeing your kitchen, your ingredients, and your meals the way chefs do.

Chefs Take Risks

One of the first keys to channeling your inner chef is to be creative. Take risks. Don't be afraid to fail. If you are used to eating the same things every day, you are a prime candidate for some creative risk taking in your food life. Remember from *Naturally Thin* the importance of variety in your diet. Risks, like using a vegetable, spice, or condiment (an accessory item) you've never tried before, nudge your palate in a new direction. You also gain confidence in your inner chef every time a risk works.

Creative ideas come by thinking about what you are doing and paying attention to the results. They come from tasting as you go and evaluating what a dish might need to taste even better. Creativity also comes from knowing your own preferences. For example, I use my immersion blender so much because I like my soups pureed. Others like their food with more texture and wouldn't use an immersion blender as much as I would.

Do you prefer bitter greens, like arugula, or the sweet, tender texture of butter lettuce? My fiancé, Jason, hates frisée and arugula and other bitter foods. I love bitter greens. Maybe you think everything is better with nuts on it. Are you a chocolate person or do you like fruity flavors more? Knowing your preferences and those of your family or guests can inspire your creativity, too. Some don't like or can't eat curry, pork, liver, or cilantro. Some people love a lot of garlic or black pepper or citrus flavors. *Know thyself.*

What's your preference? Do you love to add more vegetables? Are you all about making your meals spicy or creamy? Do you love cold foods or hot foods? Maybe you favor raw foods, or the flavors of smoked meat, or really crunchy food. *Know thyself* and you'll meet your inner chef. Spend some time thinking about your personal preferences and how those could translate to your cooking. And don't forget the six essential ingredients that I endorsed in Chapter 2: olive oil, garlic, lemon, parsley, salt, and pepper.

Another way I like to get creative with recipes is to make them into Skinnygirl recipes. I specifically look for where I can cut fat, sugar, and calories without sacrificing taste. Applying the Skinnygirl treatment has definitely resulted in some fantastic favorites, both in this book and in *Naturally Thin*. You can do this, too. Just don't change too many things in one try.

DON'T BE AFRAID

Taking risks in cooking sometimes means being willing to try things outside your comfort zone. A lot of people have very little variety in their diets, and this is often based on a fear of food. I used to eat a nonfat muffin every single day. When I went on vacation, I would obsess about whether I would be able to find one. If I didn't have one, it made me anxious. I went through another phase where I had nothing but a container of Chinese brown rice for dinner because that's what I allowed myself. People have their own special tricks or formulas or things they allow or don't allow themselves to eat, but it often comes from fear—if you break the rule, you'll go crazy, you'll eat everything, you'll get fat.

The truth is that the rules themselves can cause overeating. We naturally rebel against severe restrictions, but being in the moment instead of obsessed with rules sets you free. Now I am more in tune with my hunger and my food voice, so I eat what I'm in the mood for. Today I woke up and wanted one of the cookies I made when testing recipes for this book. That's what was in front of me, so that's what I ate. Tomorrow it might be oatmeal. The point is, now that the fear is gone, my food choices are more realistic and, as a result, they are better investments.

Chefs Have Techniques

Do you know what pan to use for what purpose? Do you know when to use high heat and when to use low heat? Do you know how to whip an egg white or fold that whipped egg white into a bowl of batter? Do you know how to get the flavor out of a garlic clove? Do you know how to make a basic soup or salad without a recipe? What about a baked potato or a bowl of rice? What do you do with ice cream? Chefs know the answers, and you can, too, after reading this chapter.

How to Boil Water (Seriously)

I'm not saying you don't know how to boil water, but I'm not assuming you do, either. If you really aren't totally sure about how to do this, then just put the amount of water you need in a saucepan or a teakettle. Turn the heat on high (one of the few times you use high heat). Cover the pan so that heat doesn't escape. The water will boil faster. When it starts to form tiny bubbles that rise to the top, that is a *simmer*. This is useful to know for soups, which often need to be simmered.

When the surface of the water has big vigorous popping bubbles, it is boiling. If it foams up out of the pan and around the lid and all over your stovetop, your water has officially boiled over. If you are paying attention, you will take the water off the heat or turn the heat down after it is boiling but before it has boiled over. If you are going to cook pasta or vegetables or something else savory in the water, add salt, add the food, bring to a boil again (the food cools down the water for a few minutes), then turn down the heat just a bit so it doesn't boil over.

How to Use Heat

Heat can make or break your cooking, so pay attention to its effects. Have you ever made pancakes and the first few were great, and then the rest of them burned? Your temperature was fine when you started, but when the skillet reached full temperature, it was too hot. Go lower next time. If your first few pancakes were too doughy and then the later ones were perfect, you started cooking before your skillet was heated all the way.

Use high heat to boil water, stir-fry vegetables, sear meat, and sear certain vegetables (like leeks and mushrooms). Never leave any food cooking on high heat for very long, and never at all if you aren't watching the pot. Otherwise, your food could burn and you could also ruin the nonstick surface on your pans. Use low heat for long-simmering dishes like soup, chili, or anything where you want to give the flavors time to develop. Low heat is also good for slowly roasting meat and for cooking rice or oatmeal. You bring it to a boil and then you reduce the heat to low and let it simmer until it is cooked.

Use medium heat as your default for everything else, but never be afraid to adjust the heat *in small increments* if you think your food isn't cooking quickly enough or is cooking too fast. This all comes with experience, but my point is that you should not be afraid to change the heat setting, even if it isn't what the recipe says.

How to Use Oil

Olive oil and butter are for use with low to medium heat. They smoke and burn on high heat. Canola oil is fine for medium and medium-high heat. If you are going to cook or fry on high heat, use peanut oil. When there is no heat involved at all—like for flavoring salads—use cold-pressed extra-virgin olive oil, sesame oil, and nut oils.

How to Deglaze a Pan

Deglazing sounds like a complicated technique, but it's not. When you sauté meat or vegetables in oil, they leave flavorful residue behind. Deglazing is a good way to use those flavors in your cooking. Let's say you sautéed onions and garlic in a pan, or chicken breast strips. After they are cooked, remove them to a plate. Leave the heat on and pour about one-quarter to one-half cup of liquid into the pan. Chefs often use wine or stock. The liquid will sizzle and immediately start to reduce, becoming more concentrated. Stir the liquid with a firm spatula or wooden spoon, loosening any bits of leftover vegetables or meat sticking to the pan. The resulting concentrated liquid can be used as a sauce over the meat or vegetables.

How to Use Salt

Salt adds flavor to foods because it enhances each ingredient's natural flavors. It's indispensable in good cooking, but you also need to know how to use it. Don't put all the salt in at the end. Then the food just tastes like bland food with salt on top of it. *Use salt as you go,* especially in soups, pasta dishes, and other foods with a lot of mixed ingredients, so that it has time to bring out the layers of flavors in your food. Even sweet foods benefit from a little salt. Don't use too much—food that is too salty is worse than food that isn't salty enough, because it's easy to add salt, but it's hard to take it away (although Chapter 5 has some tips about how to do that).

There are times when you don't want to add salt at the beginning of cooking. Foods that contain a lot of water, like mushrooms and spinach, will dry up if you salt them too early. Cook these foods first and then salt them, and they will be more tender and moist. Too much salt at the beginning can also dry out meat, so add just a little salt with lots of herbs and spices for marinating and seasoning meat before cooking, then add the final seasoning at the end.

How to Make a Salad

Salads can be boring or they can make a whole meal. You might think it's simple to make a salad, but then again, if you never like the salads you make, maybe you aren't adding the right combination of ingredients to make it special. On the other hand, if you fill a salad up with a pound of meat, cheese, and creamy dressing, you might like the taste but you know it's not a good investment, and those big salads can contain more calories than a steak dinner.

You can find a happy medium by making a great salad at home. Here's how to put one together that tastes delicious *and* is a good investment:

1. Start with leafy greens, such as mesclun mix, arugula, or baby spinach. Put a big handful into a bowl. Use about a handful for each person.
2. Add a few classic raw vegetables, such as grated carrots, sliced cucumbers, pear tomatoes cut in half, or thinly sliced red onions. Use about ½ cup, chopped, for each person.
3. Add one or two gourmet vegetables, such as a few olives, cubes of avocado, chopped artichoke hearts, roasted red peppers, or sliced hearts of palm. Use about ¼ cup for each person.

4. Add one or two special ingredients, such as a little bit of finely grated hard cheese (such as Parmesan) or crumbled cheese (such as blue cheese or feta); some dried fruit (such as cranberries or cherries); a few fresh berries (strawberries, raspberries); or a sprinkle of chopped nuts (such as sliced almonds or walnuts). About a tablespoon of each ingredient per person is plenty. You might even need a little less.

5. Drizzle with just a little bit of good dressing (such as any of the dressing recipes from this book or your favorite high-quality bottled dressing) or with extra-virgin olive oil and a squeeze of fresh lemon juice. About a tablespoon or two of dressing per person should be plenty. Toss well to combine everything. Serve and enjoy.

How to Make a Basic Vinaigrette

Store-bought salad dressing is notoriously full of chemicals. Read the label. If you see a long list of ingredients you can't pronounce, why would you want to eat that? Most commercial salad dressings are also filled with sugar.

I used to spend time making fancy salad dressings, like balsamic vinaigrette or whatever. Now, 90 percent of the time, I just dress my salads with a drizzle of olive oil, freshly squeezed lemon juice, salt, and pepper. I toss it together and it's fantastic. This is the ideal preparation when you are using high-flavor greens such as arugula and interesting additions such as avocado, hearts of palm, or artichoke hearts. These flavors stand on their own with just a little help, so you don't want to overpower them with a heavy, creamy dressing that competes with its own strong flavors. You can rarely go wrong with olive oil, lemon juice, salt, and pepper.

Salad dressing is easy to make and is a great opportunity to be creative. A classic vinaigrette is two parts oil and one part vinegar or citrus juice (acid). If you want to go lighter, you can skew those ratios, adding equal parts oil and acid, or even two parts acid to one part oil. A little bit of honey will add a nice taste—much better than adding high-fructose corn syrup like you see in many bottled commercial salad dressings. You can also add other flavoring elements. A little citrus brightens up the taste. Whenever a dressing needs a little kick, I add a dash of Worcestershire sauce.

WHAT'S A SPRIG?

Sometimes, a recipe will call for an herb sprig. These herbs grow on stiff sprigs, like little sticks, and are often used to flavor marinades. Some common examples of herbs on sprigs are thyme and rosemary. Often, they don't go into the actual dish, you take them out before you serve it. You might use them in a marinade or homemade vinaigrette.

How to Make Soup

Soup is also easy to make and a good way to use what you have. Sauté onions and/or garlic in a little bit of olive oil. When they are soft, add vegetable broth according to how much soup you want to make. Add chopped raw vegetables—whatever you have—or any frozen vegetables. Let the soup *simmer* (small bubbles) *without boiling* (big bubbles) over *medium heat* for 15 to 45 minutes. The longer soup cooks, in most cases, the better it tastes. Stir in canned beans (rinsed and drained) and/or cooked pasta about 5 minutes before you take the soup off the heat so that the beans don't fall apart and the pasta doesn't become mushy. I could tell you I soak dried beans overnight and use those, but to me the differential isn't worth it. Canned beans are fine. Don't be a hero.

At the end of cooking, adjust the liquid by adding more broth or water if the soup is too thick, then taste. If the soup is too thin, make it richer and creamier by adding a little bit of soy milk, regular milk, or yogurt. To thicken the liquid for pureed soups, a spoonful of leftover mashed potatoes or brown rice before pureeing with an immersion blender will do the trick. Add more seasonings as needed just before serving, especially salt and pepper.

How to Prepare a Protein

Don't be intimidated by the idea of sautéing, grilling, or broiling meat, fish, or tofu. It's simple. Rinse your fish, steak, chicken breast, slice of tofu, or bite-size pieces of chicken or beef, pat dry with paper towels, and heat a pan over the stove or preheat the broiler or grill. Put a thin layer of cooking oil in your pan (or on the grill), or spray it with cooking spray.

If sautéing or grilling, when the pan or grill is hot, put your protein in and sear on one side until golden brown, then flip it over *one time only*, and sear on the other side. Don't keep flipping it or it will dry out. Lower the heat and cook for a few more minutes. If you aren't sure whether it is done or not, make a cut with a sharp knife to check the center. Season with salt and pepper, remove from heat, and serve.

If broiling, put the protein in an oiled broiler pan. Cook on one side for about 5 minutes or until it starts to brown and looks cooked, then flip *once* and cook on the other side for about 5 minutes. If it's starting to get too dark, take it out and cut into it to see if it's done. Cook a little less for medium-rare, a little longer for well done.

The more you cook meat, the more you'll get a sense for how long to cook it to the degree of doneness you prefer.

Another way I like to prepare protein is to put each serving on a square of foil or parchment paper. Pat it dry and cover it with a little bit of olive oil, lemon juice, lemon zest, salt, and pepper. Wrap it up and bake at 350°F for about 30 minutes. Unwrap, save the juices to put over rice or pasta, and enjoy the succulent result—no mess. This works for any meat, poultry, fish, or tofu.

Marinating first adds more flavor. Put a little bit of citrus juice in a large plastic resealable bag or shallow pan. Add flavorings you like—olive oil, fresh or dried herbs, red pepper, black pepper, Worcestershire sauce, soy sauce, mustard, and so on. Put the protein in the marinade, turn, and let it sit for at least 30 minutes or up to overnight in the refrigerator. (Marinate fish for only 30 minutes—overnight is too long.) When you are ready to cook, take out the protein, pat it dry, and cook it in whatever way you choose.

How to Boil an Egg

I've seen a million different versions of how to do this, but it's really very easy and this version works every time: Take an egg (or more than one) and put it in a saucepan. Add just enough water to completely cover the egg. Put the pan on high heat. At the moment the water starts to boil, turn off the heat, cover the pan, and leave the pan on the burner. When the water has cooled, the egg is done. Chop up a hard-boiled egg and add a teaspoon of mayonnaise and a little bit of chopped pickle or relish, chopped celery, capers, scallions, or any other flavorings you like for a delicious egg salad. Add salt and pepper. If you want to reduce the fat, omit the yolk.

How to Make a Baked Potato

An easy way to bake a potato is to poke it all over with a fork (the holes allow steam to escape as it is baking), then rub it lightly with olive oil and salt. (If you aren't going to eat the skin, skip the oil.) Put it in an oven pre-heated to 400°F and bake until the skin is really crispy like in a fried potato-skin appetizer. This should take 45 minutes to an hour. Russet potatoes are the best kind for baking.

How to Prepare a Grain

Prepare according to package directions. For added flavor, cook in broth instead of water. Add salt, pepper, and fresh herbs or chopped fresh or frozen vegetables. Remember that different grains have different cooking times.

How to Get Corn Off the Cob

If you've ever cut corn off a cob and had the kernels fly everywhere, you probably vowed never to do it again. However, corn fresh off the cob tastes so much better than frozen that it's worth doing right. Instead of standing the cob on its end and cutting downward with your knife, put the cob flat on the cutting board, at an angle, and cut along the bottom edge with the knife parallel to the cob, turning the cob as you cut. Or, put the cob in the hole of a Bundt pan or tube pan (the round pan with the hole in the middle) and cut from there. The kernels will fall into the pan, instead of on your floor.

Beating, Whipping, Stirring, and Folding

Beating is stirring energetically in order to incorporate ingredients and change a substance's consistency. Use a fork, whisk, spoon, or electric beater.

Whipping (or whisking) is an extension of beating that incorporates even more air using a wire whisk and moving it in fast circles in your batter or egg whites. You can also do this with an electric mixer with the wire whisk attachment.

Stirring means to move ingredients around with a spatula or wooden spoon until they are incorporated so that they won't stick together (e.g., pasta or rice just added to boiling water). Stirring is more gentle and slower than beating.

ABOUT EGG WHITES AND WHIPPED CREAM

When whipping egg whites, use the wire whisk attachment on your electric mixer and whip until the eggs turn foamy and then keep getting stiffer and stiffer. Some recipes call for egg whites beaten to soft peaks, which means that when you pull out the whisk, the egg whites form peaks that flop over. Stiff peaks means the peaks stay upright when you pull out the whisk. If the recipe just says to beat egg whites until foamy, stop before they form soft peaks. *Always beat egg whites in a clean, dry bowl.* If there is any grease in the bowl, they won't transform.

To whip cream, always use a clean cold bowl and cold beaters. As you whip the cream with a wire whisk, it should approximately double in volume as it thickens. To make sweetened whipped cream, add 1 tablespoon of sugar to 1 cup of cream, with or without ½ teaspoon of vanilla or other flavoring extract. You could also add 1 tablespoon of any liqueur for a more sophisticated flavor.

Sometimes I hear about people who beat egg whites or whipped cream by hand with a wire whisk. Ow. That's not necessary.

Folding means to combine, with a spoon or preferably with a rubber spatula, from the bottom of the bowl to incorporate one kind of batter into another. This technique is common in mixing whipped egg whites into a batter. Folding is different from stirring or beating. The point is not to deflate the air pockets in something that has already been whipped or beaten, so you fold one ingredient gently over the other.

How to Get the Flavor Out of Garlic

Smash it. Literally. Put the garlic clove on a cutting board and smash it hard with the side of a chef's knife or even with a mallet. Then you can slip it right out of the skin, cut off the tips, and throw it directly into a soup, marinade, or roasted meat pan. Take the garlic clove out before serving. Its oils have flavored the dish.

If you want a stronger garlic flavor, mince it into tiny pieces or put it in a garlic press, which smashes it even further, and put the whole thing into whatever you are making.

Raw garlic has a very strong taste, but a little bit of minced raw garlic can be good in a salad dressing. A good way to prepare garlic when you will eat it raw is to mince it into very small pieces, then sprinkle it with a little salt and mash it all together with the side of your knife. The garlic and salt will turn into a paste that will dissolve in dressing and add great flavor. You can also spread this paste on bruschetta (toasted bread slices). See the recipe for Whole-Grain Bruschetta with Tomatoes and Fresh Basil (page 160).

How to Make Skinnygirl Sour Cream

Stir together 1 cup nonfat Greek yogurt and 1 tablespoon fresh lemon juice. This makes a delicious topping for a fraction of the fat and calories of regular sour cream.

How to Measure and Use Herbs and Spices

Herbs and spices add interesting flavor to so many different foods and I recommend using them liberally. You can sometimes substitute dried for fresh or fresh for dried herbs, but fresh and dried herbs have very different flavors, so keep that in mind. Generally, 1 tablespoon chopped fresh herbs equals about 1 teaspoon crumbled dried herbs.

But how do you know what herbs and spices to use? First, know what you like. The only way to discover this is by smelling and tasting. Cilantro and tarragon are two herbs with strong, unique flavors. People tend to love them or hate them, so keep that in mind when cooking for others. Some people also say they hate curry powder. I call this "curry fear." Curry is just a mixture of spices and comes in many different types, so if you think you don't like one curry you've tried, sample a different one.

If you don't think you have herbal preferences, start expanding your palate by trying different fresh and dried herbs on something that highlights their flavors. You could sprinkle different herbs on a few thin slices of French baguette, add a little olive oil, salt, and pepper, and toast them in the oven. Try each one and really pay attention to the flavor. This will help you become more adept at seasoning your foods.

Herbs and spices (and other flavoring components) can add ethnic personality to any dish. Here's how:

- For Italian flavor: oregano, basil, rosemary, garlic.
- For Latin flavor: cilantro, cumin, lime, chili, cinnamon.
- For Indian flavor: turmeric, curry, ginger, saffron, cardamom, anise, cloves, cumin.
- For Caribbean flavor: garlic, ginger, lime, allspice, cilantro, hot red peppers, Scotch bonnet peppers, coconut milk.
- For Chinese flavor: ginger, sesame seeds and oil, soy sauce, basil, garlic, five-spice powder (a spice mix), black bean sauce, hoisin sauce.
- For Japanese flavor: miso, sesame seeds, ginger, garlic, wasabi.
- For Thai flavor: Thai basil, Thai chili, curry, cumin, garlic, ginger, lemongrass, lime, tamarind, turmeric.
- For French flavor: garlic, parsley, lemon zest, tarragon, capers, herbes de Provence (a classic French herb mix containing such things as thyme, marjoram, fennel, basil, rosemary, and lavender).
- For Middle Eastern flavor: cumin, nutmeg, sumac, turmeric, za'atar (an herb mix containing things such as thyme, oregano, marjoram, sesame, and sumac).
- For Moroccan flavor: cinnamon, ginger, turmeric, saffron, paprika, dried fruits such as raisins and apricots.

How and When to Grind Spices

Black pepper is best when it's freshly ground. You can buy grinders with the pepper already in them at any grocery store. If you like to grind your own spices, the easiest way is to have a cheap coffee grinder that you use only for spices, never for coffee. You can find these for $9.99 on eBay.

However, I don't often use a grinder because I'm lazy, unless I want the spices to be very strong. Grinders are good for things like cumin and coriander seeds, but most of the time the preground spices are good enough. Don't be a hero unless the spice taste really matters in what you are making or you have the free time and the desire to grind your own. You can also grind your own nutmeg and cinnamon on your microplane, but purchased ground nutmeg and cinnamon are both just fine, too.

How to Use Ginger

Sometimes ground ginger is just fine, but freshly grated ginger has an amazing taste that you just can't quite duplicate with ground. Buy gingerroot in the produce section of the grocery store. Before you use it, peel off the hard skin on just the part you are going to use (say, one inch of the root). Then use this trick, which you won't believe until you try it: Take a regular box grater that you would use for cheese. Cover the side that grates cheese finely (the smallest holes) with plastic wrap. Grate the ginger against the plastic wrap, then pull the wrap off, and you won't have any holes in the plastic. Your ginger will be perfectly grated—just slide it off the plastic and measure it or put it right into your dish. Best of all, your grater won't need to be washed. You can also grate ginger on your microplane.

Be careful when grating less-than-fresh gingerroot because it can get fibrous and you don't want ginger fibers in your food. If your ginger looks fibrous, cut it, grate it, and just add the juice. An even easier option is to cut the ginger into a few big pieces, throw it into the dish to flavor it while it cooks, then take out the ginger pieces and throw them away before serving.

About Vanilla

If you can find and want to spend the money for a fresh vanilla bean and use the seeds in place of vanilla extract, the taste makes a difference, but vanilla beans are really pricey, so vanilla extract is fine, too. (However, do *not* use imitation vanilla extract.)

How to Make Cookies

If you are in a creative mood and you feel like making up your own cookie recipe, you can do it! All you need to remember is 1-2-3: one part sugar to two parts fat (up to half the fat could be nut butter) to three parts flour (up to one-third of the flour could be quick-cooking oats). Add whatever else you want—lemon peel, chocolate chips, walnuts, coconut, or whatever you already have in the house that you think might be good in a cookie. Add a little salt. Drop the batter by spoonfuls (or use a small ice-cream scoop) onto a baking sheet and bake at 375°F until the cookies look done, 10 to 20 minutes, depending on how big you make them. I like to use a small ice-cream scoop to portion out the cookie dough.

Part Two

What to Make:

Recipes, Conversations, and Inspiration

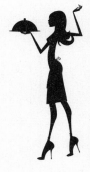

Chapter 7

Breakfast Breakthroughs

*W*hether you like to spend a lot of time or just a little on breakfast, put together something that tastes good and sets you on the right track for the day. When you dress yourself in the morning, choosing clothes that make you feel great sets the tone. It's the same with breakfast.

Some people vary breakfasts on different days and some gravitate toward different choices: hot or cold cereal; toast or some kind of bread such as a bagel or English muffin; eggs with or without some kind of breakfast meat or cheese; or something sweet like pancakes, waffles, or muffins. I talked about these various choices in *Naturally Thin*. In this book, let's talk a little bit more about how to make them in the Skinnygirl style.

Each of these typical choices can be heavy or light, depending on what you do with them. If you go light, you know you will feel better all day. I don't say that breakfast is the most important meal of the day, because all meals are important. However, making a good investment for breakfast allows you to be more decadent later. Or, you might decide that you've made such great choices so far, why blow it later? I've eaten a less-than-ideal breakfast and set a negative tone for the day, which is annoying. A good investment at breakfast is worthwhile. Within the realm of good investments, you have plenty of room for customizing your breakfast to be what you want. Let's look at some breakfast recipes that you can tailor to your own taste.

ABOUT OATS

Oats come in several types: instant or quick, old-fashioned or rolled, and steel-cut. Steel-cut oats are the least processed and the most substantial. They have a nutty, chewy texture I love. If you've never tried them, be daring and expand your horizons. If all you have in the house is rolled oats, use those. No big deal. Quick or instant oats are the most processed, but if that's easier, then that's your choice. I don't advise using the flavored packets because they are loaded with sugar (except for the plain kind), but if you are just going to have one and it's quick, it's not going to kill you.

It's a scale—not the kind you weigh yourself on (I don't believe in those) but a scale of ideal to not-so-ideal. Steel-cut oats are on the ideal end of the scale. Instant are on the other end. Just do your best and try to balance your choices throughout the day.

About Oatmeal

I eat oatmeal for breakfast occasionally, especially when I didn't have a very good dinner the night before. Oatmeal is like a blank canvas. You can add anything you like to it, and as long as you don't add *everything* you like to it, you've got a sensible and sound investment for breakfast. It's also a better choice than cold cereal, which is much more highly processed, usually includes a lot of added sugar, and is likely to make you feel hungrier sooner.

Recently I woke up realizing I needed to start my day on a good note with a good investment. I had a long photo shoot ahead of me, and I wasn't sure when I'd get to eat again or what would be available. I took a little extra time in the morning and filled up with my Love-Your-Man Steel-Cut Oatmeal recipe, full of fiber and hearty protein. I was satisfied for hours.

The basic rule for cooking steel-cut oats is to add four times as much water as oats, or water and oats at a 4:1 ratio. For old-fashioned or quick-cooking oats, you need less water because the grain is more processed and easier to penetrate, so for these add about twice as much water as oats, or water and oats at a 2:1 ratio. For example, to make two servings of steel-cut oats, add 2 cups water to 1 cup oats, or for old-fashioned/rolled oats, add 1 cup water to ½ cup oats.

Cooking steel-cut oats takes some time, so what I like to do is make a big batch, then put it in the refrigerator to last the week. Then all you have to do in the morning is microwave the portion you want. If it's too thick, add some more water while warming it up. Add some milk and dried fruit toward the end of cooking so you don't murder the fruit. Add sweetener and crunchy toppings such as nuts just before serving.

Also, remember the Brown Rice Breakfast from my first book? You can prepare other leftover grains in the same way as oatmeal, mixing in milk, dried fruit, and sweetener, and topping with nuts. For variety, try quinoa, barley, wheat, or mixed whole grains.

DAIRY AND SOY

While writing this book, I developed congestion that wouldn't go away, and my doctor said that dairy and soy could be contributing to it. I've always tried to go pretty light on dairy products, but I drink soy milk and eat soy cheese. This led me to discover some great alternatives. Now I'm experimenting with coconut milk, almond milk, and rice milk. I've also seen hemp milk, hazelnut milk, and oat milk. There are so many interesting foods out there if you look beyond the things you usually eat.

Love-Your-Man Steel-Cut Oatmeal

My fiancé looks forward to this oatmeal, so I named this recipe for him. I could just as easily have called it Love-Yourself Steel-Cut Oatmeal because it is so nourishing. Sometimes I make this and just save half for the next day. Cover it and put it in the refrigerator, then warm it up when desired.

Serves 2 (1 if you are starving)

2 cups water

½ cup steel-cut oats

2 tablespoons dried cranberries

1 tablespoon soy milk

1 teaspoon slivered almonds

2 teaspoons real maple syrup

¾ teaspoon ground cinnamon

⅛ teaspoon real vanilla extract

1. In a small saucepan, bring the water to a boil. Add the oats and reduce the heat to low. Cook for about 25 minutes, stirring occasionally.

2. Add the remaining ingredients. Cook for 5 more minutes.

~~~~~~~~~ USE-WHAT-YOU-HAVE VARIATIONS ~~~~~~~~~

Use any of these variations, or mix and match them according to your tastes.

VARIATION 1:   Instead of dried cranberries, try any other dried fruit (cherries, raisins, chopped apricots, etc.).

VARIATION 2:   Instead of soy milk, try any other plain or flavored milk (such as low-fat, coconut, almond, etc.).

VARIATION 3:   Instead of almonds, try any other chopped nut (walnuts, cashews, etc.).

VARIATION 4:   Instead of maple syrup, try any other liquid sweetener.

VARIATION 5:   Instead of vanilla extract, try any other extract (almond, orange, etc.).

VARIATION 6:   Instead of stovetop, try cooking it in the microwave. Combine
the water and oats, cover with plastic wrap or a paper towel, and cook on
50% power. Be sure you put the oatmeal in a large glass bowl or 8-cup glass
measure so that it doesn't boil over. It needs plenty of space. After it cooks, stir
in the remaining ingredients and let it sit for 2 minutes.

~~~~~~

About Pancakes

You may not have time to whip up a batch of pancakes every morning,
but on those days when you do have a little more time and you want to
just relax and enjoy the whole breakfast concept, pancakes can be perfect.
They are easy to customize with different kinds of fruits and fruit purees,
especially if you have a good solid pancake mix in your pantry. That's my
secret. Why mix together all those dry ingredients when there are excellent
pancake mixes?

I prefer multigrain mixes like the one from Arrowhead Mills. Let them
do the sifting so that you can concentrate on the pancake artistry. Pancakes
have an ideal scale, just like oats do. Whole grain flours are on the ideal end
of the scale: oat flour, buckwheat, and whole grain mixes. White flour is
on the less-than-ideal end. Just keep in mind where your choice falls on the
scale and balance it later at another meal.

If you make your pancakes from a mix, a lot of them will tell you to
add water. Instead, I like to increase the nutrient content by adding liquids
such as soy or rice milk and some fresh or dried fruit. For every serving,
use about ¼ cup of mix, about 1 teaspoon of oil, and about 6 tablespoons
of soy, rice, or skim milk. Stir in ½ cup of your favorite berries or other
chopped fruit. Top the pancakes with a little drizzle of real maple syrup, a
dusting of powdered sugar, or a couple of teaspoons of your favorite jam.

Another good way to think ahead is to make a batch of pancakes, have
two, and put the rest into individual containers with two pancakes and two

pieces of veggie or turkey sausage. Now you've got microwavable breakfasts for the week. Don't be afraid to do this. Your pancakes don't have to be made that morning. Weight-loss meal delivery services often include pancakes for breakfast and you can be sure those weren't made that same day. If they can do it, so can you.

Like all the other recipes in this book, this one contains lots of variations so that you can make it yours. It was originally published in my *Health* magazine column, "Celebrity Diet Secrets."

Whole-Grain Blueberry Pancakes

I lightened up a basic blueberry pancake recipe for Trista Sutter (former star of *The Bachelorette*) her husband, Ryan, and their children.

Serves 3

¾ cup multigrain pancake mix
   (such as Arrowhead Mills)
1 tablespoon canola oil
⅓ cup plus 2 tablespoons soy
   milk

½ cup fresh blueberries
Topping: A little bit of real
   maple syrup, powdered
   sugar, or jam

1. Combine the pancake mix, canola oil, and soy milk in a bowl and stir until just combined. The batter can be a little lumpy. Spray a nonstick griddle or skillet with cooking spray and place over medium heat. Pour six pancakes onto the griddle or skillet, using about ¼ cup of the batter (or use a 2-ounce ice-cream scoop) for each pancake. Sprinkle with a few blueberries.

2. Cook over medium heat for 2 to 3 minutes or until the tops are covered with bubbles and the edges look cooked. Flip the pancakes over and cook for an additional 2 to 3 minutes, or until the bottoms are golden brown. Stack the pancakes on a plate and cover with a clean hand towel to keep them warm. Drizzle or sprinkle on the topping when you serve.

Use any of these variations, or mix and match them according to your tastes.

VARIATION 1: Instead of multigrain pancake mix, try any other whole-grain or gluten-free pancake mix. Or, make your own with ¾ cup oat flour or other whole-grain flour, 1 teaspoon baking powder, and ¼ teaspoon salt.

VARIATION 2: Instead of soy milk, try any other plain or flavored milk.

VARIATION 3: Instead of blueberries, try any other fresh or frozen berries or other chopped fruit, such as peaches or apples.

VARIATION 4: Try adding any of the following:
~ 1 or 2 tablespoons chopped nuts ~ 1 or 2 tablespoons mini–chocolate chips ~ 1 or 2 tablespoons unsweetened coconut ~ ½ teaspoon ground cinnamon ~ ¼ cup pumpkin or butternut squash puree.

About Eggs

Sometimes I want eggs for breakfast. Maybe I didn't get enough protein the night before, or maybe I had one too many Skinnygirl Margaritas. Whatever the reason, when I wake up craving eggs, you can bet I'll make them.

Eggs are an excellent source of protein, but I'm not going to eat a four-egg omelet with a pound of cheese and bacon and turn the whole meal into a disaster. I like mine with just a sprinkle of cheese. Maybe you like yours with some salsa and green onions or sautéed mushrooms and a little bit of chopped turkey bacon. I don't have eggs every day, but when I do, I enjoy them. Eggs are a great canvas for ingredients, too. Look at restaurant menus and all the different things they put into omelets. Borrow some of those ideas if you want to make your eggs more exciting. Don't be afraid to try something new.

I always use the finely shredded cheese or I grate it myself on a microplane for a very fine grate. The "regular" shredded cheese comes in big, fat shreds. It's too much. The finely shredded cheese allows you to add just a tiny bit and still enjoy the taste and experience of cheese.

Perfect Scrambled Eggs

I make great scrambled eggs. It's one of my things. When I make scrambled eggs, I use a very basic formula: two eggs. That's it. No milk, no water, no club soda, no separating out the egg whites. My secret for cooking them is to turn the stove on high. Use a nonstick skillet and let it get really hot. Spray it lightly with olive oil or canola oil cooking spray, add the eggs, stir once, and *turn off the heat*. The pan will already be very hot and will cook the eggs exactly right so that they aren't too runny and they aren't too hard. Stir until they're cooked, then serve immediately. Some people might tell you that cooking eggs over high heat will make them too tough. I have never had this experience. Because I turn off the heat as soon as I add the eggs, they turn out perfect, so don't be afraid to try this.

You also might wonder about the whole eggs. I would rather eat two whole eggs than three times the amount of egg substitute, but if the *differential* is small for you and you like egg whites, you could make this with one egg and two egg whites or even with all egg whites (use four).

Serves 1

2 eggs
Salt and pepper to taste

1 to 1½ teaspoons finely
shredded cheese

1. Put a nonstick skillet on the stove and turn the heat to high. Let the pan get very hot. Meanwhile, break the eggs into a small bowl and beat them lightly with a fork or a wire whisk.

2. Spray the pan with cooking spray. Add the eggs and stir once. Turn off the heat. Sprinkle with a little salt and pepper. Leave the pan on the burner and continue stirring until the eggs are cooked. The residual heat will cook the eggs.

3. Sprinkle the eggs with the cheese and serve. Perfect!

~~~~~~~~ USE-WHAT-YOU-HAVE VARIATIONS ~~~~~~~~

Use any of these variations, or mix and match them according to your tastes.

VARIATION 1:   Try adding leftover vegetables, vegetable combinations, fresh herbs, or a spoonful of salsa.

VARIATION 2:   Try adding extra protein, such as:
~ 1 slice Canadian bacon, chopped ~ 1 slice turkey bacon, crumbled
~ 1 slice veggie bacon, crumbled ~ 1 vegetarian sausage patty or link, chopped.

VARIATION 3:   Substitute the cheese with any other crumbled or shredded cheese, including nondairy cheese.

Make this recipe vegan by using 3 ounces extra-firm drained tofu instead of the eggs. Pat it dry and toss it with 1 teaspoon soy sauce. Use medium-high heat instead of high. Crumble the tofu into the hot oiled pan and stir constantly until it gets golden and crispy.

~ ~

About French Toast

If I'm going to eat scrambled eggs, I'm going to eat the whole egg, but for something like an omelet with a lot of added ingredients or for French toast, there isn't a whole lot of point to eating the yolk because egg whites give you the same effect. It's the differential again.

Whole-Grain French Toast

French toast is really simple and even quicker to make than pancakes. It's also thrifty because it's a good way to use up bread that's a little stale. Stale bread works best because it doesn't fall apart. I also like to make this recipe using sprouted grain bread like Ezekiel because it is naturally dense and doesn't get mushy when it soaks in the egg mixture. My new favorite way to make French toast is to use the Pepperidge Farm Deli Flats which are just 100 calories each.

Serves 2

4 egg whites
1 teaspoon real vanilla extract
1 teapsoon maple syrup
4 slices any whole-grain bread,
  preferably slightly stale

Topping: Real maple syrup
and/or fresh fruit

1. In a shallow pan big enough to hold four slices of bread, combine the egg whites, vanilla extract, and maple syrup. Beat lightly with a fork or a wire whisk. Put the four slices of bread into the pan, then flip them over to coat both sides.

2. Spray a nonstick skillet or griddle with cooking spray and place over medium heat. Remove the bread from the pan, mopping up any leftover egg whites with the bread. Cook the slices in the preheated skillet for 2 to 3 minutes on each side.

3. Serve immediately, drizzled with a small amount of maple syrup and topped with your favorite fresh fruit. (If you don't have fresh fruit, heat ½ cup frozen fruit and serve it warm. This is nice in the winter when fresh fruit isn't in season.)

~~~~~~~~ USE-WHAT-YOU-HAVE VARIATIONS ~~~~~~~~

Use any of these variations, or mix and match them according to your tastes.

VARIATION 1:   Instead of whole-grain bread, try sprouted-grain bread, sourdough bread, or Pepperidge Farm Deli Flats.

VARIATION 2:   Instead of vanilla extract, try any other flavored extract.

VARIATION 3:   Instead of maple syrup, try any other liquid or dry sweetener.

VARIATION 4:   Instead of the maple syrup topping, try:
~ A spoonful of jam ~ 1 teaspoon mini–chocolate chips per serving ~ A spoonful of whipped cream ~ A sprinkle of powdered sugar.

~~~~~~

About Muffins

Muffins are easy to buy at any bakery or Starbucks, but beware. Those big, delicious, cakey muffins are about the same as eating cake, with the same calorie and fat content. If you can buy them and eat half, that might work for you on some days. A better investment is to make your own at home and bring them with you. You can keep homemade muffins in the freezer and grab one on your way to work. By the time you get there, it should be defrosted. Or, take one out the night before so that it's ready to eat in the morning.

When you make your own muffins, you control the ingredients and the size. A basic muffin recipe is all you need. Then you can customize it to include your favorite ingredients, from applesauce to Zante currants.

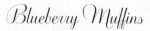

Blueberry Muffins

This muffin recipe is great. You can substitute other fresh fruit for the blueberries.

Makes 6 to 8 muffins

1¼ cups oat flour

¾ cup raw sugar

1½ teaspoons baking powder

¼ teaspoon salt

½ cup soy milk

2 tablespoons trans-fat-free shortening, melted

¾ teaspoon real vanilla extract

¾ cup fresh blueberries

1. Preheat the oven to 350°F. Line a cupcake or muffin pan with liners.

2. Combine the flour, sugar, baking powder, and salt in a bowl. In another bowl, combine the soy milk, melted shortening, and vanilla extract.

3. Add the wet ingredients to the dry ingredients and mix until just combined. Stir in the blueberries.

4. Using an ice-cream scoop, drop the batter into the muffin liners. Bake for 20 minutes, rotating the pan after 10 minutes so that the muffins cook evenly. When done, the muffin tops should be firm. Let them cool for at least 15 minutes and serve warm or at room temperature.

~~~~~~~~ USE-WHAT-YOU-HAVE VARIATIONS ~~~~~~~~

Use any of these variations, or mix and match them according to your tastes.

VARIATION 1: Instead of oat flour, try any other flour, preferably whole grain.

VARIATION 2: Instead of raw sugar, try any other dry granulated sweetener.

VARIATION 3: Instead of soy milk, try any other plain or flavored milk.

VARIATION 4: Instead of vegetable shortening, try butter (regular or nondairy) or any cooking oil.

VARIATION 5:   Instead of vanilla extract, try any other compatible extract.

VARIATION 6:   Instead of blueberries, try any other berry or chopped seasonal fresh or frozen fruit; any canned, drained, rinsed fruit; or any fruit puree.

VARIATION 7:   Make this recipe sweeter and a little more decadent by adding a tablespoon or two of mini–chocolate chips or any chopped nut.

~ ~

Skinny Quiche

I skinnified this quiche for *Gossip Girl*'s Kelly Rutherford.

Serves 6

1 store-bought whole-grain
   frozen pastry shell, such as
   Wholly Wholesome brand
2½ teaspoons olive oil, divided
2 shallots, thinly sliced
1 package (about 5 ounces)
   prewashed fresh baby
   spinach
½ teaspoon salt, divided

¼ teaspoon black pepper
1 package (4 or 5 ounces)
   assorted mushrooms
⅔ cup freshly grated Parmesan
   cheese
1 cup soy milk
1 egg
3 egg whites

1. Preheat the oven to 375°F. Bake the pastry shell for 12 minutes or until browned. Remove the shell from the oven and set aside. Leave the oven on.

2. Heat 1¼ teaspoons of the olive oil in a large nonstick skillet over medium heat. Add the shallots and sauté for 1 minute. Add the spinach and cook for 2 to 3 minutes, or until wilted. Add ¼ teaspoon of the salt and a dash of pepper. Transfer to a plate and set aside.

3. Using the same pan, heat the remaining olive oil and cook the mushrooms for about 6 minutes, stirring occasionally, until they are browned on both sides. Remove from the heat. Season them with the remaining salt and pepper.

4. Sprinkle ⅓ cup of the Parmesan cheese over the bottom of the pastry crust. Top with the spinach and mushroom mixtures. In a separate bowl, whisk together the soy milk, egg, and egg whites. Pour into the shell, over the spinach and mushrooms. Top with the remaining Parmesan.

5. Bake the quiche for 45 to 50 minutes, or until the top is firm and golden brown. Cut into wedges and serve hot or warm; or make ahead, refrigerate, and serve cold.

~~~~~~~~~ USE-WHAT-YOU-HAVE VARIATIONS ~~~~~~~~~

Use any of these variations, or mix and match them according to your tastes.

VARIATION 1:   Instead of a frozen pastry shell, try:
~ A refrigerated pastry shell that you unfold and bake ~ A homemade piecrust, if you like to make it ~ No crust—just spray the pie pan with cooking spray first, or assemble in individual ramekins or muffin tins. These effectively become frittatas.

VARIATION 2:   Instead of olive oil, try any other cooking oil or butter.

VARIATION 3:   Instead of shallots, try any onion or onion substitute (leeks, scallions, or chives).

VARIATION 4:   Instead of the fresh baby spinach, try any other favorite fresh chopped cooking greens or ½ cup frozen, defrosted, well-drained spinach.

VARIATION 5:   Instead of the mushrooms, try any other fresh or frozen defrosted vegetable, such as:
~ Broccoli rabe ~ Asparagus ~ Artichoke hearts ~ Sliced red bell pepper ~ Diced tomatoes.

VARIATION 6:   Instead of the Parmesan, try any other crumbled, grated, or shredded cheese, or even no cheese.

VARIATION 7:   Instead of the soy milk, try any other plain unflavored milk.

VARIATION 8:   Try adding extra protein, such as:
~ 1 slice Canadian bacon, chopped ~ 1 slice turkey bacon, crumbled
~ 1 slice vegetarian bacon, crumbled ~ 1 vegetarian sausage patty or
link, chopped.

~~~~~~

Chapter 8

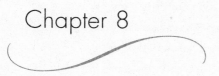

Light Lunches

I don't always get the time to sit down to a good lunch, but when I do, I don't like to eat heavy food or I'll be tired and dragging through the afternoon. With these light yet substantial and satisfying lunches, you'll be able to face the afternoon feeling nourished and energized, not bloated and tired.

This chapter is divided into three sections, for when you want a sandwich, soup, or a salad for lunch. I'm not saying you have to eat soup, salad, or sandwiches for lunch, and in fact, any of the dinner recipes in this book would be fine for lunch, too. However, I've focused on these quick and easy lunch items in this chapter because if you are like me, you usually don't have a lot of time for lunch.

If you make these recipes the night before, you can have a lunch packed and ready to go with you to work. *Note:* There are a few recipes in this chapter that I renovated for various celebrities. Those originally appeared in my column in *Health* magazine, in a slightly different form.

About Sandwiches, Wraps, and Burgers

Throw tasty ingredients between two slices of bread or roll them up in a tortilla and you've got a hearty, satisfying lunch. There is nothing wrong with including two slices of fiber-rich, nutrient-dense bread with your lunch, no matter what the carb haters say. (Don't get me started on the whole low-carb fiasco.) Or one slice—no one says you can't have just half a sandwich if that's all you want or you aren't particularly hungry.

When you do have a whole sandwich, just realize that you have had two slices of bread and watch your starch intake at the next meal. A sandwich-for-lunch day is not the day to have pasta for dinner. Save pasta for your soup-and-salad days. That's how you balance your diet like a bank account. That being said, I recently had a fattening lobster salad sandwich with mayonnaise, avocado, cheese, and two pieces of bread because I really wanted it. I enjoyed it, but I reeled it in at the next meal.

About Bread

What's a sandwich without bread? Your choice of bread can make or break your sandwich. Choose carefully, because some breads are such a racket, masquerading as real food. They say "wheat" on the package, but they are really just beige-colored white bread. It's a bunch of BS. Store-bought bread is typically very highly processed and made with mostly white flour that just makes you hungrier. It's like you didn't even eat anything.

Like many kinds of food, there is an ideal scale for bread. White bread is at the not-ideal end. Grainy, dark bread and sprouted-grain bread are at the ideal end. All the other kinds of bread exist somewhere in between, so keep that in mind when making your choice.

Personally, I prefer sprouted-grain bread because it doesn't contain any flour, so it's less processed. It's a high-volume, fiber-rich bread that is filling and nutritious with a delicious nutty taste and chewy texture. It makes me appreciate that I'm actually eating something. A good bread investment is more than a frame. It's something good you are doing for yourself.

Food for Life makes excellent sprouted-grain products, including one of my favorites, Ezekiel bread. It's widely available. You may be able to find other brands or local versions in your supermarket or health food store.

THE SCOOP

All bagels, English muffins, and sandwich buns can easily be "scooped." In case you don't remember from *Naturally Thin,* scooping is what I do to lighten up a big, thick chunk of bread. I just pull out some of the bread in the middle of the English muffin, bagel, or bun, which also makes more room for the filling. You get all the bread enjoyment while cutting the calories. If you are concerned with wasting that filling, just keep it in a plastic resealable bag in the freezer for the next time you need bread crumbs. To be totally truthful, sometimes when I'm really hungry, I eat the scooped bagel, then I butter the part I scooped and eat that, too. Just do the best you can. It's fine.

If you can't find sprouted-grain bread, at least look for breads that are made with whole grains, like whole-wheat bread and multigrain bread. They will usually be darker, coarser, more substantial, and heavier, with more fiber. Look for breads that have a rough texture, dark color, and show the grains and seeds. I'm also fond of the new Pepperidge Farm Deli Flats for sandwiches because they are just 100 calories and come in wheat, 7-grain, and oat flavors. Because they are so thin, you don't need to scoop them.

Another good option is sourdough bread. It looks like white bread, but it's a better choice than white bread. It has a tangy flavor and chewy texture that makes a sandwich more interesting.

If white bread is your only choice, just remember to balance it. Can you make up for that white-bread investment in some other way? (Is it worth skipping dessert?) Just know that you are getting a lot less fiber.

About Veggies

Sandwiches are a great way to add more vegetables to your diet. So many different kinds of raw vegetables taste good on a sandwich, like to-mato slices, arugula, spinach, cucumber slices, shredded carrots . . . I could go on and on, but I'm sure you can use your imagination to think of more possibilities. At every sandwich opportunity, try to add some kind of raw vegetable. You can also mix raw vegetables into tuna or chicken salad to add volume and fill you up. Look for good ways to add fiber and volume to your tuna or chicken salad.

About Spreads

Spreads can add intense flavor to a sandwich, or they can triple the fat content, so watch the spreads. If you like mayonnaise, try the dairy-free or low-fat kind. Personally, I think the *differential* between regular and low-fat mayonnaise is nothing. Sometimes I like to cut my mayo with mustard to lower the fat even more, while adding mustard flavor. A homemade dijon-naise is delicious on a sandwich—just mix a teaspoon of mayo with a tea-spoon of Grey Poupon (or your favorite brand).

Mashed avocado (or guacamole) makes a delicious rich spread, but pick your fat. Don't use avocado and mayonnaise and cheese (like I did when I ate that lobster sandwich! Just do your best.) Pick the one you want most. You can always make a different choice next time. Remember, *you can have it all, just not all at once.* Other good spreads are hummus, tapenade, and pesto. A little sprinkle of extra-virgin olive oil and good vinegar or fresh lemon juice can also make a sandwich more interesting. The slight sprinkle of oil you will get from this kind of topping comes to hardly any fat but a lot of flavor.

For burgers, try mixing ketchup with mustard. Ketchup is fine in small amounts, but it often contains high-fructose corn syrup, which is one of the most processed sweeteners you can buy (check your ketchup label). There are health food versions of ketchup that use other sweeteners, but they are all different forms of sugar. Know what you are eating. If you prefer your sandwiches spicy, try Asian chili sauce or chipotle mayo.

Considering these Skinnygirl pointers, eat what you want. A half sandwich is usually plenty for me if I also have a cup of soup or a small salad. If not, I eat the whole sandwich, and if you want to, you should, too. Here are some of my favorite sandwich recipes, plus ways to make them your own.

Mykonos Burger

I revised this recipe for Maria Mykonos. It might not be authentically Greek, but it calls up those flavors and it's a lot of burger for a small calorie price.

Serves 4

1 pound lean ground turkey

⅓ cup plus 1 teaspoon (for yogurt sauce) chopped fresh parsley plus more for garnish

¾ teaspoon freshly ground black pepper plus more for yogurt sauce

½ teaspoon salt plus more for yogurt sauce

1 tablespoon Worcestershire sauce

1 tablespoon Dijon mustard

½ teaspoon garlic powder

1¾ ounces crumbled feta cheese

4 whole-wheat hamburger buns, toasted

4 slices (about ¼ inch thick) red onion

½ cup Greek yogurt

½ teaspoon lemon juice

1. In a medium bowl, combine the ground turkey, parsley, pepper, salt, Worcestershire sauce, mustard, garlic powder, and feta cheese. Use an ice-cream scoop or ½-cup measure to make 4 equal-size patties.

2. Put the patties on a broiler pan lined with foil and sprayed with cooking spray. Broil the patties for 5 to 6 minutes on each side, or until done.

3. Place each burger on the bottom half of a bun. Top with the onion slices. In a medium bowl, combine the yogurt, 1 teaspoon parsley, lemon juice, salt, and pepper. Top the burgers with the sauce and garnish with more parsley, if desired. Cover with the top half of the bun.

Use any of these variations, or mix and match them according to your tastes.

VARIATION 1:   Instead of ground turkey, try any other ground meat, or mixture of ground meats, or a veggie burger (cook as directed on the package and just add toppings).

VARIATION 2:   Go Asian with this burger instead of Greek.
Instead of Worcestershire sauce, try soy sauce or Wasabi mayonnaise.

Cut the garlic powder to ¼ teaspoon and add ¼ teaspoon ground ginger.

Instead of parsley, try Thai basil or cilantro.

Instead of feta cheese, try ½ cup shiitake mushrooms sautéed in 1 teaspoon sesame oil.

Instead of topping with red onion and yogurt sauce, try:
~ Raw Napa cabbage leaf ~ Asian slaw ~ Sweet and sour sauce.

VARIATION 3:   Go Latin with this burger instead of Greek.
Instead of Worcestershire sauce, try chipotle sauce.

Cut the garlic powder to ¼ teaspoon and add ¼ teaspoon chili powder.

Instead of parsley, try cilantro.

Instead of feta cheese, try any sharp cheese like Monterey Jack or any crumbled or shredded Mexican cheese.

Instead of topping with red onion and yogurt sauce, try:
~ Pickled jalapeños ~ Red or green salsa ~ 1 slice of avocado or a spoonful of guacamole.

VARIATION 4:   Instead of serving these burgers on buns, serve them:
~ On toasted English muffins ~ On toasted bagels ~ On toasted Pepperidge Farm Deli Flats.

~~~~~~

Cranberry Almond Chicken Salad

This recipe was born from the leftover Boyfriend Roast Chicken (page 130). I was sitting around with my assistants and we wanted to make chicken salad out of the leftovers. I happened to have almonds. I thought of raisins but didn't have any, so I added cranberries. Somehow those things together seemed autumnal to me, so I took a risk and added some cinnamon, which I normally wouldn't do. Happy accident! It was a delicious risk.

If I had happened to have cashews instead of almonds, maybe I would have thought to add golden raisins, and that would have made me think of curry powder. I've never (yet) made chicken salad with cashews, golden raisins, and curry powder, but because I've seen things like this in delis, it probably would have occurred to me based on what I had. This is what I mean when I say to pay attention to the way restaurants and delis put together food—it gives you ideas and can spark the creative process.

I like this salad because it is a meaty, deli-style salad without the calories and fat of the old-school mayo-filled variety. Serve it on whole-grain toast with romaine lettuce leaves and tomato slices.

Serves 2

1 cup shredded cooked chicken
(leftover or even good-
quality canned)
1 tablespoon slivered almonds
1½ tablespoons dried cranberries
1½ tablespoons nondairy
mayonnaise

Pinch of cinnamon
½ teaspoon Dijon mustard
½ teaspoon salt
½ teaspoon black pepper

Combine all of the ingredients in a bowl and mix well.

Use any of these variations, or mix and match them according to your tastes.

VARIATION 1:   Instead of chicken, try shredded turkey or any other cooked poultry.

VARIATION 2:   Instead of almonds, try any other chopped nut or any seeds.

VARIATION 3:   Instead of dried cranberries, try:

~ Raisins ~ Currants ~ Chopped dried apricots.

VARIATION 4:   Instead of nondairy mayonnaise, try any other mayonnaise.

VARIATION 5:   Instead of cinnamon, try:

~ A dash of nutmeg ~ 1 tablespoon chopped fresh dill ~ 1 tablespoon chopped fresh basil ~ ½ teaspoon dried rosemary.

VARIATION 6:   Instead of Dijon mustard, try any other flavored or plain mustard, such as spicy, cranberry, horseradish, etc.

~~~~~~

Mozzarella, Arugula, and Sun-Dried Tomato Panini

A panini is really just a flattened-out version of a grilled sandwich, in the spirit of grilled cheese, but it is traditionally cooked on the top and the bottom at the same time on a grill. Panini makers or presses are inexpensive and worth the money if you make panini a lot. They are like those George Foreman grills and they give you the classic grill marks. The presses cook the panini quickly, they are versatile (you can cook a lot of different things in them—I sometimes use them to grill tofu slices), and they are also very easy to clean. I like Breville's panini press.

However, you don't need a panini press to make panini. Assemble your sandwich, lightly brush it with oil, and put it in a hot nonstick skillet. Put a sheet of aluminum foil over the sandwich and put a heavy pan on top (cast iron works well) to press it down while it is cooking. When the bottom side is golden brown, remove the top pan, flip the sandwich, and repeat on the other side. If you have a grill pan, use that to get the characteristic panini grill marks. You can also make panini on the barbecue with a brick wrapped in aluminum foil. Incidentally, bricks are also good for grilling meat on its own, in the style of dishes like "chicken under a brick."

Serves 4

8 slices whole grain bread

¼ cup olive oil

8 thin slices mozzarella cheese

2 cups arugula

16 sun-dried tomatoes, soaked
    in warm water for 10
    minutes and cut into thin
    strips

½ cup chopped fresh basil

½ teaspoon garlic powder

Salt and pepper to taste

1. Preheat the panini maker or heat a nonstick skillet over medium heat.

2. Brush one side of one piece of bread with olive oil. Top with one slice of cheese, one-quarter of the arugula, one-quarter of the sun-dried tomato strips, one-quarter of the basil, and a sprinkle of garlic powder, salt, and pepper. Top with a second slice of cheese and a second slice of bread. Brush the top of the bread with olive oil and put the sandwich between the plates of the panini maker or onto the skillet and cover with a piece of foil and a second heavy skillet.

3. When the light on the panini maker goes on, remove the sandwich and repeat to make four sandwiches. If you aren't using a panini maker, use a spatula to keep an eye on the underside of the sandwich. When it is golden brown, flip and cook the other side, then remove the sandwich and repeat. The time this takes will vary according to the heat of your skillet, so watch the panini carefully to avoid burning.

Use any of these variations, or mix and match them according to your tastes.

VARIATION 1:   Many types of bread work in a panini maker. Instead of whole-grain bread, try your favorite bread, preferably whole grain. You might try foccacia, sourdough baguette, or Pepperidge Farm Deli Flat.

VARIATION 2:   Instead of mozzarella, try any other crumbled, shredded, or sliced cheese.

VARIATION 3:   Instead of arugula, try your favorite leafy salad greens.

VARIATION 4:   Instead of sun-dried tomatoes, try one or more of the following: ~ Sliced olives ~ Chopped marinated artichoke hearts ~ Fresh tomato slices.

VARIATION 5:   Instead of fresh basil, try any other fresh leafy herb.

VARIATION 6:   For even more vegetable goodness and volume, add any grilled leftover vegetables you happen to have.

VARIATION 7:   For more protein, add any thinly sliced poultry or beef.

VARIATION 8:   For even more flavor, try adding: ~ A drizzle of olive oil and herb or balsamic vinegar ~ A squeeze of fresh lemon juice ~ Dijon mustard ~ Hot sauce ~ Flavorful spreads like pesto, tapenade, or hummus.

~~~~~~

Tuna on Whole-Grain Bread

Sometimes I just want a tuna salad sandwich. I like mine pretty basic with soy mayo and fresh herbs, but if you like to fill your tuna salad with extras, see the list of variations for ideas. Extra veggies always add nutrients and volume to tuna salad, so the more, the better. As for that notion that half or a third of a can of tuna is enough . . . huh? I don't know about you, but I almost always eat the whole can. To make just one serving, cut this recipe by one-fourth.

Serves 4

4 cans (about 6 ounces each)
    white tuna in water, drained
½ cup nondairy mayonnaise
2 teaspoons Dijon mustard
⅓ cup chopped fresh parsley

¼ cup chopped fresh dill
Salt and pepper to taste
8 slices bread
4 slices nondairy cheese

1. In a bowl combine the tuna, mayonnaise, mustard, parsley, and dill. Season with salt and pepper.

2. Spread the tuna mixture on 4 slices of the bread, add the cheese, and top with the final slice of bread for each sandwich.

~~~~~~~~~ USE-WHAT-YOU-HAVE VARIATIONS ~~~~~~~~~

Use any of these variations, or mix and match them according to your tastes.

VARIATION 1:   Instead of tuna, try:
   ~ 2 Cups shredded or chopped cooked chicken ~ 2 cups chopped cooked shrimp ~ 8 hard-boiled eggs, mashed with a fork (or leave out some of the yolks) ~ 2 pounds extra-firm tofu, drained and crumbled.

VARIATION 2:   Instead of nondairy mayonnaise, try low-fat mayonnaise, or Greek yogurt.

VARIATION 3:   Instead of parsley and/or dill, try any other fresh herb.

VARIATION 4:   Instead of salt and pepper, try your favorite seasoning salt.

VARIATION 5:   For more flavor, try adding:
   ~ Capers ~ Chopped black or green olives ~ Chopped roasted red peppers ~ Pickle relish or chopped pickles.

VARIATION 6: For more volume and nutrients, try adding any chopped raw vegetables, such as celery, carrots, or bell peppers.

VARIATION 7: Serve this salad over mixed greens and skip the bread.

VARIATION 8: Instead of nondairy cheese, try thin slices of any other cheese.

~ ~

GIVE YOUR MAYO PERSONALITY

Sometimes I like plain mayonnaise, but sometimes, I want to make my mayo more exciting. You can add so many different flavors to mayonnaise to match whatever kind of sandwich you are having. Add any of the following to ½ cup regular or soy mayonnaise (enough for about 4 sandwiches):

- 1 tablespoon chopped chipotle peppers in adobo sauce, for a Latin flavor
- 1 tablespoon minced sun-dried tomatoes, chopped olives, or tapenade, for a Mediterranean flavor
- 1 tablespoon barbecue sauce
- 1 tablespoon pesto
- 1 teaspoon soy sauce
- ½ teaspoon prepared horseradish
- ½ teaspoon Old Bay or Cajun seasoning, for a New Orleans–inspired flavor
- ½ teaspoon curry powder, for an Indian flavor
- ½ teaspoon wasabi or grated fresh ginger, for an Asian flavor
- 1 teaspoon Worcestershire sauce, for zest
- 1 tablespoon chopped fresh herbs, for a fresh flavor

Sandwiched Leftovers

What did you have for dinner last night? What do you have in the refrigerator that you need to eat? Can you make it into a sandwich today? There are so many options, so take this basic concept and run with it. Here are some ideas to use as inspirations for your own sandwich creations:

- Slices of steak with arugula and sliced tomato in a whole-grain wrap with a thin spread of mayonnaise.
- Shredded or chopped chicken mixed with curry powder, low-fat mayonnaise, chopped green apples, chopped celery, walnuts, salt, and pepper stuffed into a toasted whole-wheat pita.
- Turkey slices with avocado, tomato, sprouts, baby spinach, and mustard on a toasted, scooped whole-grain bun.
- If you order salad in a restaurant and you know you won't eat it all, just put dressing on half of it and get the rest to go. Without dressing, it will stay fresher so that you can use it the next day. Roll your leftover Caesar, chef's, or Cobb salad into a whole-grain tortilla or stuff it into a toasted pita. If you are making a wrap, get a 6- or 10-inch whole-grain tortilla. That's plenty for most people. Even the tortillas that say they are "burrito size" can be too big for lunch.
- Put leftover hummus, bean dip, or guacamole on toast and top it with mixed greens, tomato, cucumbers, carrots, and a drizzle of vinaigrette. Eat it with a fork.

~~~~~~~~ USE-WHAT-YOU-HAVE VARIATIONS ~~~~~~~~

Use any of these variations, or mix and match them according to your tastes.

FIRST: Pick your bread. Any bread will work, preferably whole-grain, including English muffins, bagels, and wraps.

SECOND: Pick your filling, according to what you have left over:
  ~ Steak ~ Chicken ~ Turkey ~ Grilled tofu ~ Roasted vegetables.

THIRD: Pick your spread:

~ Soy or regular mayonnaise ~ Guacamole or mashed plain avocado
~ Mustard ~ Greek yogurt with dill and chopped cucumbers ~
Baba ghanoush ~ Ratatouille ~ Hummus ~ Sun-dried tomato pesto ~
Tapenade.

FOURTH: Pick your toppings:

~ Leafy greens ~ Chopped or sliced raw vegetables ~ Flavor zips, like
olives or artichoke hearts ~ Any cheese.

FIFTH: Put it all together and enjoy.

~ ~

About Soup

I'm a huge fan of soup. It fills you up and provides concentrated nutri-
tion without a lot of fat and calories. You know I don't mean creamy soups
like New England clam chowder or potato cheese soup. However, once you
learn my tricks, you'll even be able to renovate the fattening ones. But most
of the time, the best, healthiest, most filling soups are those made from
broth and vegetables, pureed or chunky, including vegetable soups, noodle
soups, and bean or pea soups.

You can make soup out of just about any vegetable. I don't always make
my own because some brands of canned soups, like Amy's, are quick, taste
good, and take no time to make. I also like some of the healthy boxed soups,
like those made by Pacific and Imagine. Even brands like Campbell's are
now making good boxed soups, like butternut squash. If you can pronounce
and comprehend most of the ingredients, go ahead and enjoy a canned or
boxed soup. When you have a little more time, soup is easy to make and a
great way to use what you have. Try these soups I like to make, or make
them your own way using the variations.

White Bean with Spinach Soup

This easy soup fills you up and tastes so satisfying that you might not need anything else, but it's also good with a salad or half a sandwich or with just a small slice of crusty bread.

Serves 4

1 teaspoon olive oil

1 yellow onion, thinly sliced

1 clove garlic, smashed

½ red bell pepper, minced

4 cups vegetable broth

1 can white beans (about 15 ounces), drained and rinsed

2 cups chopped fresh baby spinach

1 bay leaf

½ teaspoon salt plus more if needed

½ teaspoon pepper plus more if needed

1. In a nonstick pot, heat the olive oil over medium-high heat. Add the onion and sauté until it softens, about 5 minutes. Add the garlic and bell pepper and sauté until the pepper softens, about 5 more minutes.

2. Add the vegetable broth, white beans, spinach, bay leaf, salt, and pepper. Simmer for about 20 minutes, or until the soup is hot. Remove the bay leaf and the garlic with a slotted spoon and throw them away.

3. Puree the soup with an immersion blender until it is completely smooth (the way I like it), or leave some of the beans chunky, if you prefer some texture. Taste and add more salt and pepper if necessary. Serve hot.

~~~~~~~~ USE-WHAT-YOU-HAVE VARIATIONS ~~~~~~~~

Use any of these variations, or mix and match them according to your tastes.

VARIATION 1:   Instead of red bell pepper, try any other color bell pepper.

VARIATION 2:   Instead of vegetable broth, try chicken broth.

VARIATION 3:   Instead of white beans, try:

~ Black-eyed peas ~ Chickpeas ~ Lima beans.

VARIATION 4:   Instead of fresh baby spinach, try ½ cup frozen defrosted
spinach, drained or any other chopped cooking green (like kale,
chard, etc.).

VARIATION 5:   For more flavor, try adding:

~ 1 teaspoon dried oregano ~ 1 teaspoon dried rosemary ~
1 tablespoon fresh basil.

~ ~

Carrot Ginger Soup

This spicy-sweet-gingery soup has a lot of character and it goes well with an
Asian salad or with a sandwich. It freezes well so you can make a batch on the
weekend and put it in individual containers to reheat during the week.

Serves 4

*1 teaspoon butter (regular or
    nondairy)*
1 teaspoon olive oil
*2 cloves garlic, peeled and
    minced*
1 tablespoon grated fresh ginger
1 yellow onion, chopped
½ teaspoon ground cumin
½ teaspoon ground coriander

4 cups chicken broth
½ cup dry white wine
Juice and zest from 1 lemon
*2 cups chopped or shredded
    carrots*
Salt and pepper to taste
*4 tablespoons chopped fresh
    parsley*

1. In a nonstick pot over medium-high heat, combine the butter and olive
oil. When the butter has melted, add the garlic. Sauté until just beginning to turn

golden, about 5 minutes. Add the ginger, onion, cumin, and coriander. Sauté until the onion gets soft, about 5 more minutes. Add the chicken broth, white wine, and lemon juice and zest. Stir to combine. Add the carrots.

2. Bring the mixture to a boil and then immediately lower the heat to a simmer. Cook until the carrots are very soft, 30 to 45 minutes (test them by piercing them with a fork—it should go through the carrots easily). Taste and add salt and pepper as needed.

3. Using an immersion blender, puree the soup until it is smooth. Taste again and adjust the salt and pepper as needed. If you want an even smoother texture, strain it through a fine mesh strainer. Serve hot topped with chopped parsley.

~~~~~~~~ USE-WHAT-YOU-HAVE VARIATIONS ~~~~~~~~

Use any of these variations, or mix and match them according to your tastes.

VARIATION 1:   Instead of olive oil, try any other cooking oil.

VARIATION 2:   Instead of garlic, try 1 teaspoon garlic powder.

VARIATION 3:   Instead of yellow onion, try any other onion, 2 leeks, or
4 shallots.

VARIATION 4:   Instead of cumin and coriander, try 1 teaspoon curry powder or
½ teaspoon each turmeric and paprika.

VARIATION 5:   Instead of chicken broth, try any other broth, stock, or water.

VARIATION 6:   Instead of carrots, try:
~ Any cubed, shredded, or cooked and pureed winter squash (like butternut or acorn) ~ Any potato (sweet or white), peeled and cut into cubes ~ 2 cups pumpkin puree (not pumpkin pie mix).

VARIATION 7:   Instead of parsley, garnish with chopped fresh cilantro.

~~~~~~

Sweet Tomato Soup

This recipe involves a little bit of chopping, so this might justify breaking out the food processor. It's totally vegan even though it's creamy and sweet, so enjoy! This recipe goes quickly if you chop and measure all your ingredients before you start putting it all together. If you chop everything well enough, you won't have to puree this soup, but you can if you prefer a really smooth tomato soup. If you like tradition, serve this with a grilled cheese sandwich (use any cheese, including nondairy) or with any panini described earlier in this chapter.

Serves 4

1 tablespoon olive oil

1 yellow onion, finely chopped

2 stalks celery, finely chopped

1 clove garlic, minced

3 carrots, finely chopped

1 bay leaf

½ cup tomato paste

1 pound fresh tomatoes, diced (save the juices)

4 cups vegetable broth

½ teaspoon salt plus more if needed

½ teaspoon black pepper plus more if needed

2 tablespoons oat flour

½ cup soy milk

2 tablespoons raw sugar

Zest and juice from 1 lemon

1 teaspoon apple cider vinegar

1 teaspoon chopped fresh dill

1. In a nonstick pot, heat the olive oil on medium-high heat. Add the onion and sauté until soft, about 5 minutes. Add the celery and garlic and sauté for 5 more minutes. Add the carrots, bay leaf, tomato paste, tomatoes, vegetable broth, salt, and pepper. Bring the soup to a boil, then lower the heat to medium-low and let it simmer for 20 minutes.

2. In a small bowl, whisk together the oat flour and soy milk until smooth. Stir into the soup and let it simmer for 10 more minutes.

3. Rinse out that small bowl and add the sugar, lemon zest and juice, and vinegar. Stir together until the sugar dissolves. Add this mixture to the soup. Let the soup simmer for 5 more minutes, then taste. Add more salt and pepper if necessary. Remove the bay leaf. Serve hot sprinkled with fresh dill.

~~~~~~~~ USE-WHAT-YOU-HAVE VARIATIONS ~~~~~~~~

Use any of these variations, or mix and match them according to your tastes.

VARIATION 1:   Instead of yellow onion, try any other onion, 2 leeks, or 4 shallots.

VARIATION 2:   Instead of fresh tomatoes, try a can (about 15 ounces) of fire-roasted diced tomatoes.

VARIATION 3:   Instead of vegetable broth, try any other broth or stock, or water.

VARIATION 4:   Instead of oat flour, try any other flour.

VARIATION 5:   Instead of soy milk, try light coconut milk or any other milk.

VARIATION 6:   Instead of raw sugar, try any other dry or liquid natural sweetener (honey, maple syrup, etc.).

VARIATION 7:   Spice your soup up even more by adding any one of the following:
~ 1 teaspoon any dried herb (like oregano or thyme) ~ ½ teaspoon any savory spice (like paprika, turmeric, or cumin) ~ ¼ teaspoon any ground sweet spice (like nutmeg or cinnamon) ~ ¼ teaspoon red pepper flakes ~ Dash of hot sauce ~ Swirl of pesto ~ Swirl of lowfat sour cream ~ A few avocado slices ~ A few tortilla strips.

~~~~~~

About Salads

I don't eat raw vegetables every day, even though it would be great if I did. Sometimes I just don't have a chance and sometimes I'm just not in the mood. However, I try. I want you to try, too, because raw vegetables are so full of nutrients. Raw vegetables are more difficult to eat in the winter when you are more likely to want something warm like soup but in summer, crisp cold salads are the ultimate lunch. Even so, some salads can be heartier and more warming with ingredients like corn, avocados, nuts, or warm chicken.

Salads are a great way to use what you have because the greens provide a fresh crunchy background for meat, chicken, fish, grilled vegetables, beans, or whatever you feel like eating. Salads can be made out of so many different ingredients that they are one of the easiest ways to start practicing your creativity. Here are some of my favorite recipes to get you started. When you get in the salad habit, you will actually find yourself craving vegetables. That's when you know you really are living the Skinnygirl lifestyle.

Arugula Salad with Simple Dressing

I think this easy, colorful salad is the world's perfect dish. Because the arugula is so flavorful, it only needs a simple dressing. I love arugula, but use any leafy green *you* love. *Always* lightly salt your salad greens.

Serves 2 as an entrée, 4 as a side salad

6 cups arugula (I like baby arugula for this salad)
1 ear raw corn kernels (yes, raw—you will become addicted to the sweet flavor)
1 avocado, halved, pitted, scored into cubes, and removed with a spoon

⅔ cup pear tomatoes cut in half (or use cherry or grape tomatoes)
Salt and pepper to taste
Fresh basil cut in thin strips, for garnish

Arrange the arugula on a platter. Sprinkle the corn on top, then arrange the avocado pieces and tomatoes over the corn. Season with salt and pepper and drizzle the Simple Dressing (see following recipe) over the salad. Garnish with basil.

Simple Dressing

This recipe looks too simple, but trust this dressing. Some of the best things are amazingly simple. The first time I dressed a salad with lemon juice, olive oil, salt, and pepper, it was a revelation.

Juice from 1 small lemon
2 tablespoons extra-virgin olive oil
Salt and pepper to taste

Whisk all of the ingredients together in a bowl and taste. If the dressing is too puckery for you, add a drizzle of honey.

~~~~~~~~ USE-WHAT-YOU-HAVE VARIATIONS ~~~~~~~~

Use any of these variations, or mix and match them according to your tastes.

VARIATION 1: Instead of arugula, try any dark leafy green, such as:
~ Baby spinach ~ Mesclun greens ~ Watercress ~ Arugula.

VARIATION 2: Instead of fresh raw corn, try ½ cup frozen defrosted corn, well drained, or ½ cup fresh or frozen defrosted peas, well drained.

VARIATION 3: Instead of avocado, try:
~ ½ cup chopped hearts of palm ~ ½ cup chopped canned or jarred artichoke hearts, well drained ~ ½ cup canned garbanzo beans, rinsed and drained.

VARIATION 4: Instead of pear tomatoes, try any other fresh tomato.

VARIATION 5: In the dressing, instead of lemon juice, try any other citrus juice.

~ ~

Asian Shrimp Salad

This filling entrée salad makes an excellent lunch as well as an elegant side salad when you have guests for dinner. If you have precooked and deveined shrimp or leftover shrimp from dinner the night before, it takes just minutes to prepare.

Serves 8 as an entrée, 12 as a side salad

1 package (about 5 ounces) prewashed fresh baby spinach

1 medium head Napa cabbage, shredded

1 pound sugar snap pea pods, halved

1 small can (about 6 ounces) water chestnuts, drained and sliced

1 cup shredded carrots

1 pound cooked chilled shrimp, split in half lengthwise (16 to 20 count)

1 bunch scallions, chopped, green parts only

4 ounces sliced toasted almonds (toast them in a skillet over medium heat, stirring constantly, for about 5 minutes)

Toss all of the ingredients together in a bowl and serve with the following Asian Dressing recipe.

Asian Dressing

This dressing also makes an excellent marinade for meat or fish. If you aren't in the mood to make dressing (although this is really easy), Newman's Own has an excellent low-fat Asian vinaigrette. It's organic and it's good, and I'd rather you spend your time getting really nice, fresh spinach and cabbage and other vegetables. It's up to you and how much time and energy you have.

2 teaspoons grated fresh ginger

4 teaspoons dark sesame oil

¼ cup rice vinegar

4 teaspoons soy sauce

2 teaspoons Dijon mustard

2 teaspoons minced garlic

6 tablespoons extra-virgin olive oil

Whisk all of the ingredients together in a bowl.

~~~~~~~~ USE-WHAT-YOU-HAVE VARIATIONS ~~~~~~~~

Use any of these variations, or mix and match them according to your tastes.

VARIATION 1: Instead of spinach, try your favorite leafy salad greens.

VARIATION 2: Instead of Napa cabbage, try any shredded cabbage or small bag (about 7 ounces) of coleslaw mix.

VARIATION 3: Instead of sugar snap peas, try:
~ Fresh raw or cooked peas ~ Frozen defrosted peas ~ Fresh or frozen defrosted French green beans, chopped.

VARIATION 4: Instead of water chestnuts, try canned baby corn, drained, or hearts of palm, chopped.

VARIATION 5: Instead of shrimp, try shredded chicken or chopped or cubed steak.

VARIATION 6: Instead of almonds, try any other chopped toasted nut.

VARIATION 7: In the dressing, instead of grated ginger, try ½ teaspoon ground ginger or ½ teaspoon Chinese five-spice powder.

VARIATION 8: Instead of rice vinegar, try any other vinegar or citrus juice.

VARIATION 9: Instead of extra-virgin olive oil, try any other good-quality cold-pressed oil (sesame, safflower, etc.).

~ ~

MIX AND MATCH

I won't touch fat-free dressings. I hate them. To me they taste like sugary, disgusting chemical glue. But I can't bring myself to douse my salad in 200 calories of fat, either. When a salad calls for a creamy, ranch-style dressing, I've found that the perfect solution is to mix light ranch dressing with a light vinaigrette in a 1:1 ratio, for all the ranch flavor with a fraction of the fat.

Healthier Cobb Salad

Cobb salads give salad a bad name. In many restaurants, this salad is just a big pile of bacon, chicken, blue cheese, hard-boiled eggs, avocado, and ranch dressing over a little bit of lettuce. I don't even want to think about how much fat is in a typical Cobb salad and dressing at a restaurant. I'm not mad at Cobb salad—I order it sometimes and eat a small quantity. However, what I love about the Cobb salad is that it was originally invented to use up leftovers. If you love the Cobb salad taste and you want to lighten it up, try this recipe. It's quick and easy when you've got leftover chicken and turkey bacon—and, of course, you can always make your own version, according to what leftovers *you* have. Nothing says it absolutely has to be chicken and bacon. And for the dressing, try the ranch and vinaigrette combination that I recommend.

Serves 8 as an entrée, 12 as a side salad

6 hearts of romaine, chopped
1 small package turkey bacon (about 6 ounces) cooked in the microwave until crisp and crumbled
Shredded white meat from a purchased 2-pound rotisserie chicken
2 pints pear tomatoes, halved or quartered

10 ounces Danish blue cheese (Danablu), crumbled
3 avocados, halved, pitted, scored into cubes, and removed with a spoon
5 hard-boiled egg whites, coarsely chopped
¾ cup purchased low-fat ranch dressing or half low-fat ranch mixed with half light vinaigrette

Arrange the romaine on plates or on a serving platter. Arrange the salad ingredients in stripes over the lettuce, then drizzle the dressing in stripes over the top.

~~~~~~~~ USE-WHAT-YOU-HAVE VARIATIONS ~~~~~~~~

Use any of these variations, or mix and match them according to your tastes.

VARIATION 1: Instead of romaine, try any crispy leafy salad green.

VARIATION 2: Instead of turkey bacon, try:
~ Chopped Canadian bacon ~ Crumbled veggie bacon ~ Chopped lean ham ~ Smaller amount of regular bacon (about 4 ounces).

VARIATION 3: Instead of chicken, try any chopped, shredded, or cubed beef, poultry, shrimp, or tofu.

VARIATION 4: Instead of pear tomatoes, try any other kind or color of tomato.

VARIATION 5: Instead of blue cheese, try any strongly flavored crumbled or shredded cheese.

VARIATION 6: Instead of avocados, try 1 cup chopped artichoke hearts, or 1 cup sliced hearts of palm.

VARIATION 7: Instead of hard-boiled egg whites, try ½ cup crumbled extra-firm tofu.

VARIATION 8: Instead of low-fat ranch mixed with light vinaigrette, try: ~ ½ cup low-fat ranch mixed with a squeeze of fresh lemon juice, salt and pepper, and ¼ cup water ~ Light vinaigrette only ~ A drizzle of olive oil and fresh lemon juice seasoned with salt and pepper.

~ ~

Chapter 9

Delicious Dinners

I love dinner, although I don't always get a chance to have dinner. Dinner is when most people sit down, unwind, relax, and really enjoy good food and each other. Dinner is your fabulous evening outfit, whether it's simple and classic or head-turning. Dinner is how you make an impression, not just on your family and your guests, but on yourself. It's a chance to shine. When it comes to eating at home and having the time to actually go in the kitchen and make something, dinner is where it happens. I always want you to pay attention and savor your food, tasting every bite. You probably have more time to do this at dinner than you do for other meals. The world doesn't always stop for breakfast or lunch, so dinner is worth a little effort.

I don't mean cooking effort, though. None of these recipes are what I would call difficult. These are minimalist recipes, just like the rest of the recipes in this book—quick and easy to make with ingredients you probably already have on hand or can easily pick up at the market. They are made with accessorized classics. These recipes are just a base for your own experimental creations so that you can make the dinner you love without feeling like you've overdone it. As with the last chapter, some of these recipes first appeared in my column in *Health* magazine, where I renovate favorite foods of different celebrities.

Family-Friendly Dinners

Other chapters in this book include recipes that might appeal to a more mature palate. For those of you with families, rest assured that all the recipes in this chapter are pretty family-friendly. Maybe your kids don't like vegetables *now,* but try these recipes on them and start exposing them to vegetables of all kinds when they are young and you'll raise a house full of vegetable lovers.

I don't have kids, so take my advice with a grain of salt, but I used to be a kid and I've dated people with small children. It's my impression that kids are pretty coddled these days when it comes to food. We hand them special menus with hot dogs and cheeseburgers or we make special meals of pizza or macaroni and cheese for them instead of encouraging them to eat what the adults are eating. Is it really their fault that they don't like vegetables or more interesting flavors? You can't take teenagers raised on pepperoni pizza and suddenly start shoving eggplant and arugula on their plates.

However, you can start to make more gradual changes in your family's eating habits, toward more variety, more vegetables, and more exotic flavors—and less fat and sugar. So your kids don't want the dinner you prepared? Trust me, they aren't going to starve. We aren't in Ethiopia. Give your kids a shot at a healthy future. I was eating escargot at the age of four and sushi in fifth grade. I never knew what a kids' menu was, and I think my palate is more developed as a result. Granted, I've had to overcome a lot of food noise, but that's why I can now look back and see what went wrong. I suppose one good thing about my childhood was the fact that I was never given any special meals just because I was a child. It's just something to think about if you have kids.

I do understand that a lot of kids are picky eaters. With that in mind, the entrée recipes in this chapter are mostly familiar dishes made in a more healthful way, so kids won't think they are weird. You won't, either (a lot of adults are picky eaters, too).

Boyfriend Roast Chicken

I developed this recipe because I had a date with the guy who is now my fiancé. We had been dating for a while, but I hadn't cooked for him yet. I wanted to impress him and make dinner a cozy, intimate experience. I wanted to spend time with him, not with my stove, so I chose something that I didn't need to babysit. I wanted to serve comfort food, and nothing says comfort like a nice golden-brown chicken with crispy skin. Whoever said the path to a man's heart is his stomach was wise.

It was the end of winter and still chilly outside, so I also thought of roasted vegetables and sweet potatoes. I had recently bought one of those soup starter kits from the produce department. It had carrots, turnips, and onions, so those are the vegetables I roasted. This is another example of using what you already have on hand. I happened to have green beans and some almonds, so I made those, too. The soup kit also had celery and fresh dill, so I used those to jazz up the salad.

If you know you are going to roast a chicken, buy fresh herbs when you buy the chicken. Fresh herbs don't keep for very long, so it's good to buy them right before you need them. You can always use the leftovers in a salad or soup. I used the leftover chicken from this recipe in two different salads that you can find in Chapter 8.

1 roast chicken, 3 to 3½ pounds

Salt and pepper to taste

1 yellow onion, cut in half

½ carrot

½ stalk celery

½ lemon

2 cloves garlic, smashed

2 sprigs each fresh rosemary,
thyme, and oregano

1 tablespoon olive oil

1 tablespoon melted butter

1. Preheat the oven to 350°F. Rinse the chicken and pat it dry. If the chicken has the giblets or neck inside, remove those and lightly season the inside of the chicken with salt and pepper. Put half the onion, carrot, celery, lemon, garlic, and fresh herbs inside the chicken. Tie the legs together with twine. Slice the remaining onion and put it in a roasting pan sprayed with cooking spray. Put the chicken on this bed of onions.

2. In a small bowl, combine the olive oil and melted butter. Using a basting brush, brush every inch of the chicken with the olive oil–butter mixture. Season the entire chicken with salt (or garlic salt) and pepper and bake on the middle oven rack for 1 hour and 15 minutes.

3. Turn up the oven temperature to 375°F and cook for another 30 to 45 minutes, or longer if your oven isn't as hot or your chicken is a little bigger. If the top still isn't crispy, put the chicken under the broiler for a few minutes to completely brown it. You will know the chicken is done when you pull at the leg and it feels ready to come off and the juices run clear (not pink) when you pierce the skin with a knife.

4. Remove the chicken from the oven and cover it with foil in a loose tent shape. Let it sit for about 20 minutes so that the juices can settle into the meat, then serve with any of the vegetable side dishes in this chapter. Remember to use what you have.

Use any of these variations, or mix and match them according to your tastes.

VARIATION 1:   Instead of salt, try any seasoning salt, such as garlic salt.

VARIATION 2:   Instead of yellow onion, try any other onion, 4 shallots, 10 pearl onions, or 2 leeks, coarsely chopped.

VARIATION 3:   Instead of the carrot, try ½ turnip, chopped, or ½ parsnip, sliced.

VARIATION 4:   Instead of celery, try chopped fennel or bok choy.

VARIATION 5:   Instead of lemon, try any citrus juice.

VARIATION 6:   Instead of garlic, try ½ teaspoon garlic powder or ½ teaspoon garlic salt (reduce other salt in this recipe).

VARIATION 7:   Instead of fresh rosemary, thyme, and oregano, try ½ teaspoon each dried rosemary, thyme, and oregano, or sprigs of any other fresh herbs you have, like parsley, cilantro, tarragon, or savory.

VARIATION 8:   Instead of olive oil and melted butter, try any other cooking oil, melted nondairy or regular butter, or any combination of liquid fats.

~~~~~~

Mashed Sweet Potatoes

This is great comfort food and a versatile recipe you can use later in other things, so if you have leftovers, that's great. Think ahead about other things you might want to do with this dish. You could add some beaten egg whites to the leftovers and bake them as a soufflé (you can find the recipe on page 216). You could use leftovers in muffins or a pie instead of canned pumpkin. You could add the leftovers to pancake batter. Or, save the skins, restuff them with the mash, sprinkle with cinnamon-sugar mixture, and bake them as twice-baked sweet potatoes.

Serves 4 to 6

4 small sweet potatoes or yams (whichever is brighter in color), peeled and chopped into large chunks
Salt to taste
2 tablespoons unsalted butter (regular or nondairy)

2 tablespoons soy milk
1 tablespoon honey
1 teaspoon salt
¼ teaspoon ground cinnamon
⅛ teaspoon scooped seeds from a real vanilla bean
⅛ teaspoon ground nutmeg

1. Put the potatoes in a large pot of cold salted water. Turn the heat to high and heat until the water starts boiling, then reduce the heat to medium to avoid splattering. Cook the potatoes until they are tender when you pierce them with a fork.

2. Drain the potatoes in a colander, then put them in a large bowl. Add all of the other ingredients and combine with a potato masher. Once you've got most of the lumps out, puree with an immersion blender to make the potatoes completely smooth. Taste and add salt if needed. Serve hot.

~~~~~~~~ USE-WHAT-YOU-HAVE VARIATIONS ~~~~~~~~

Use any of these variations, or mix and match them according to your tastes.

VARIATION 1:   Instead of sweet potatoes, try any peeled, cubed winter squash (acorn, pumpkin, butternut, etc.) or frozen, defrosted winter squash puree.

VARIATION 2:   Instead of soy milk, try:
~ Any other plain unflavored milk ~ Low-fat regular or nondairy sour cream
~ Buttermilk ~ Any plain yogurt ~ Reduced-fat or nondairy sour cream.

VARIATION 3:   Instead of honey, try any other dry or liquid sweetener.

VARIATION 4:   Instead of or in addition to ground cinnamon, try

⅛ teaspoon dried cardamom or ⅛ teaspoon ground allspice. Note smaller amounts, as these spices are more intense than cinnamon.

VARIATION 5:   Instead of vanilla bean seeds, try ¼ teaspoon real vanilla extract.

~~~~~~

Roasted Winter Vegetables

These are deliciously comforting, ridiculously easy, and a great way to use up any root vegetables you have in your refrigerator. This dish is nutrient-dense, too, with very little fat—a good complement to any roasted meat. Leftovers are great the next day over brown rice or chopped and added to mixed greens for a salad. Add fresh parsley for bright green against the muted color of the roasted vegetables. This dish is like dressing up a gray dress with hot red pumps.

Serves 4

1 parsnip, peeled and chopped into bite-size pieces

1 turnip, chopped into bite-size pieces

2 medium red potatoes, peeled or not, chopped into bite-size pieces

1 carrot, peeled and chopped into bite-size pieces

Leaves from 6 sprigs fresh thyme

1 tablespoon olive oil

¾ teaspoon salt

½ teaspoon black pepper

1 teaspoon chopped fresh parsley

1. Preheat the oven to 375°F. Cover a roasting pan or sheet pan with foil, to minimize cleanup.

2. Toss all of the ingredients except the parsley together in a bowl (or directly in the roasting pan). Bake until soft yet slightly crispy on the outside, 30 to 45 minutes (depending on how big you cut the pieces). Sprinkle with fresh parsley before serving.

Use any of these variations, or mix and match them according to your tastes.

VARIATION 1:   Instead of parsnips, turnips, potatoes, and carrots, substitute equivalent amounts of any combination of winter squash or other firm vegetables (tender vegetables will get too mushy), such as butternut squash, zucchini (thickly sliced), broccoli/cauliflower florets, and onions.

VARIATION 2:   Instead of fresh thyme, try:
~ 1 tablespoon any other chopped fresh herb ~1 teaspoon any crumbled dried herb.

VARIATION 3:   Instead of olive oil, try any other cooking oil or melted nondairy or regular butter.

VARIATION 4:   Instead of salt, try any seasoning salt.

VARIATION 5:   Instead of fresh parsley, try any other fresh leafy herb.

~ ~

Almond Green Beans

This recipe is really easy. If you don't have fresh green beans, frozen are okay as long as they are very well defrosted and drained, but aren't quite as good as fresh. Don't use canned, though. They are just too mushy. You have to draw the line somewhere. Cook these until they are the texture you like. Just keep tasting.

¼ cup slivered almonds

1 tablespoon olive oil

1 pound fresh green beans,
*   tough ends trimmed (cut*
*   them off with a knife or just*
*   snap them off with your*
*   fingers)*

1 teaspoon fresh lemon juice

¾ teaspoon salt

½ teaspoon black pepper

1 tablespoon salted butter
*   (regular or nondairy)*

1. Toast the almonds in a nonstick pan over medium heat, stirring constantly until they start to turn golden brown and smell toasted. Remove from the heat and set aside.

2. Heat the olive oil in a large nonstick pan on high heat. Add the beans, lemon juice, salt, and pepper. Sauté for 5 minutes, then turn down the heat to low. Cover the pan and continue to cook until the beans are steamed yet crispy, about 5 more minutes or a little longer, depending on the thickness of the beans. Toss with the butter, sprinkle with the crispy toasted almonds, and serve hot.

~~~~~~~~ USE-WHAT-YOU-HAVE VARIATIONS ~~~~~~~~

Use any of these variations, or mix and match them according to your tastes.

VARIATION 1: Instead of slivered almonds, try any other chopped nut.

VARIATION 2: Instead of olive oil, try any other cooking oil or melted nondairy or regular butter.

VARIATION 3: Instead of green beans, try:
~ Sugar snap pea pods ~ Sliced zucchini ~ Broccoli rabe or broccolini ~ Asparagus.

VARIATION 4: Instead of fresh lemon juice, try any citrus juice.

~~~~~~

Healthy Tacos

Tacos are quick, fun, and easy to put on the table, and so many ingredients can become taco filling that this is an almost indispensable meal when you have to feed more than just yourself. Even if it's just you, almost anything you had for dinner last night can probably be made into taco filling. Meat, veggies, cheese . . . it all works.

"Regular" tacos can be a greasy mess of fried meat, lard-filled beans, and fatty cheese. That's not how Skinnygirls eat. Plus, the problem with crunchy taco shells is that they are fried. If they ever come out with whole-grain baked taco shells, I'll be on board, and one fried taco shell is not going to make you gain 5 pounds overnight. However, I prefer soft tacos because you can buy low-fat whole-wheat tortillas. They have more fiber and more volume. Warm them in the microwave and let everyone put the ingredients they like on their own taco. With this recipe, all the ingredients are good investments, so no matter what people choose, they'll be getting a good meal.

Serves 4

1 pound lean ground turkey

2 teaspoons chili powder

2 teaspoons ground cumin

1 teaspoon garlic salt

1 teaspoon black pepper

1 teaspoon paprika

1 teaspoon Worcestershire
  sauce

½ teaspoon Tabasco sauce

½ teaspoon Dijon mustard

¼ teaspoon red pepper
  flakes

4 whole-wheat tortillas

Toppings (such as ¼ heart
  romaine lettuce, shredded ~
  ½ cup shredded reduced-
  fat cheddar cheese ~
  ½ cup shredded reduced-fat
  Monterey Jack cheese ~
  Skinnygirl sour cream (1 cup
  nonfat Greek yogurt mixed
  with 1 tablespoon fresh lemon
  juice)

1. Spray a nonstick skillet with cooking spray and put over medium heat. Crumble the ground turkey into the pan. Add the next nine ingredients and cook, stirring and breaking up the meat with a wooden spoon or spatula, until the meat is browned. Set aside.

2. Wrap the tortillas in a towel and heat in the microwave for 15 to 30 seconds. To serve, put the meat, tortillas, and toppings on serving plates. Everyone can make their own taco.

~~~~~~~~ USE-WHAT-YOU-HAVE VARIATIONS ~~~~~~~~

Use any of these variations, or mix and match them according to your tastes.

VARIATION 1:   Instead of ground turkey, try:
Any ground or shredded meat or poultry ~ Cooked shrimp ~ Refried beans ~ Veggie crumbles ~ Canned black beans, drained and rinsed.

VARIATION 2:   Instead of chili powder, try:
Taco seasoning mix ~ Cajun seasoning mix ~ 1 tablespoon prepared salsa or taco sauce.

VARIATION 3:   Instead of garlic salt, try any regular or seasoned salt.

VARIATION 4:   Instead of Worcestershire sauce, try:
~ Soy sauce ~ Tamari ~ Fish sauce (for shrimp tacos).

VARIATION 5:   Instead of Tabasco sauce, try any other hot sauce.

VARIATION 6:   Instead of red pepper flakes, try cayenne pepper or chili powder.

VARIATION 7:   Instead of or in addition to the toppings listed, try:
~ 1 fresh tomato, chopped, mixed with 1 or 2 scallions, chopped, with or without a little bit of chopped fresh or pickled jalapeño pepper ~ Chopped fresh cilantro ~ Red or green salsa ~ Chopped iceberg lettuce ~ Any other sharp cheese, Mexican cheese, feta cheese, or goat cheese ~ Guacamole or avocado slices.

~~~~~~

Healthier Baked Ziti

I'm not going to eat a pound of pasta in one sitting, but I love pasta and I eat it often. Whole grain pasta in a sensible serving size is a great investment and an important staple to keep in your pantry at all times. If you have the basics, you can always make this delicious, savory comfort food.

Whenever I make pasta with sauce, I always use pasta rigate, which means the pasta has ridges. The ridges hold the sauce to the pasta. On smooth shapes, the sauce tends to slide off.

When you split a pound of pasta between four people, that's enough for a main-course serving. Add a salad and maybe an additional side dish like roasted asparagus or sautéed broccoli and you've got a complete dinner. By the way, this is a great dish to bring to a potluck.

I always try to add vegetables to pasta dishes. It stretches out the pasta—you can eat more food and get more fiber and nutrients with less starch.

Serves 4

16 ounces whole-wheat ziti

15 ounces part-skim ricotta cheese

½ cup freshly grated Parmesan cheese

1 teaspoon garlic salt

¾ teaspoon freshly ground black pepper

1 egg white, lightly beaten

2 cups tomato sauce

8 ounces shredded fresh part-skim mozzarella cheese, (the kind you buy in a tub of water—drain it well before using)

2 tablespoons chopped fresh parsley

2 tablespoons chopped fresh basil

1. Preheat the oven to 350°F. Cook the ziti according to the package directions until still slightly firm, or about 8 minutes. You don't want to overcook the pasta because it will cook more in the oven. If you have a soup pot that can go

FRESH VERSUS DRIED PASTA

I usually use dried pasta, just because it is easier to store and because its firm texture goes well with hearty sauces. However, fresh pasta can have a place in your refrigerator, too, if you plan to eat it right away. Fresh pasta has a softer texture and tastes delicious with a lighter sauce or with just a little butter and fresh herbs. Try them both to get a sense of the difference. Recently, I've seen whole-wheat fresh pasta, which is a great option.

directly into the oven, use that. Otherwise, while the pasta is cooking, spray a casserole with cooking spray.

2. Drain the ziti and return it to the pot. Let it cool. In a separate bowl, mix the ricotta, Parmesan, garlic salt, black pepper, and egg white. When the ziti is about room temperature, stir the ricotta mixture into the ziti until everything is combined. Stir in the tomato sauce and mozzarella.

3. If you are using a casserole, pour the mixture into the casserole. Or, leave it in the oven-proof pot. Bake uncovered for 20 minutes. Serve warm.

~~~~~~~~ USE-WHAT-YOU-HAVE VARIATIONS ~~~~~~~~

Use any of these variations, or mix and match them according to your tastes.

VARIATION 1:   Instead of ziti, try any other short, stubby pasta (preferably whole-grain).

VARIATION 2:   Instead of tomato sauce, try a can of tomatoes (about 15 ounces), pureed in the blender.

VARIATION 3:   Instead of ricotta, try part-skim cottage cheese, whipped or not, or silken tofu.

VARIATION 4:   Instead of fresh mozzarella, try:
~ Farmer's cheese ~ Soy mozzarella ~ Provolone.

VARIATION 5: Instead of Parmesan, try any other highly flavored grating cheese, such as Romano or Pecorino.

VARIATION 6: Instead of garlic salt, try any regular or seasoned salt.

VARIATION 7: Leave out the egg white.

VARIATION 8: Instead of parsley and/or basil, try any combination of:
~ Thyme ~ Rosemary ~ Oregano.

~ ~

My Healthy Version of Pad Thai

For the first six months that my former assistant Molly worked for me, she ordered pad thai every day. It's a great comfort food, but the problem with most restaurant versions is that they are very high in fat, sugar, and starch, and it's easy to over-stuff yourself on the noodles. I decided I needed to create a Skinnygirl version, reducing the oil and eliminating the egg, which doesn't seem necessary to me. When I developed this recipe, I used what I already had in my kitchen. Molly loved this version. (And she lost 30 pounds!)

Serves 4

1 package (about 14 ounces) Asian rice noodles (the flat, wide, linguine-shaped kind, sometimes called pad thai noodles)

1 tablespoon soy sauce or tamari

1 clove garlic, minced

½ teaspoon chili paste

½ teaspoon minced fresh ginger

½ teaspoon fish sauce

½ teaspoon honey, warmed so that it is soft

½ teaspoon fresh lime juice

¼ teaspoon toasted sesame oil

¼ teaspoon salt

¼ teaspoon black pepper

2 tablespoons chopped fresh cilantro

1½ tablespoons chopped cashews

1. Cook and drain the rice noodles according to the package directions. Set aside.

2. In a small bowl, combine the soy sauce, garlic, chili paste, ginger, fish sauce, honey, lime juice, sesame oil, salt, and pepper. Whisk until blended and pour over the noodles. Toss to coat, top with the cilantro and cashews, and serve warm.

~~~~~~~ USE-WHAT-YOU-HAVE VARIATIONS ~~~~~~~

Use any of these variations, or mix and match them according to your tastes.

VARIATION 1:   Instead of rice noodles, try any other Asian or regular long noodle, preferably whole-grain, such as soba noodles, linguine, or angel-hair.

VARIATION 2:   Instead of chili paste, try chili powder, chili oil, or any hot sauce or chili sauce.

VARIATION 3:   Instead of fresh ginger, try ¼ teaspoon ground ginger.

VARIATION 4:   Instead of fish sauce, try additional soy sauce or tamari.

VARIATION 5:   Instead of honey, try any other natural liquid sweetener.

VARIATION 6:   Instead of fresh lime juice, try any other citrus juice.

VARIATION 7:   Instead of toasted sesame oil, try any other cooking or cold-pressed oil, including flavored oils like chili oil, or nut oils.

VARIATION 8:   Instead of or in addition to cilantro, try:
~ Chopped fresh Thai basil or regular basil ~ Bean sprouts ~ Grated or thinly sliced Napa cabbage.

VARIATION 9:   Instead of cashews, try any other chopped nut.

~~~~~~

Game-Time Zesty Baked Chicken Wings

These aren't like buffalo wings with a lot of sauce. These are flavorful, zesty, lemony wings baked instead of fried in oil, making them an excellent investment. The chicken marinates for a few hours. Since you don't need to babysit it, you can do other things. Actual prep time is quick. These wings are good to serve with the Zesty, Cheesy Mac and Cheese (from *Naturally Thin*) or any light pasta dish such as the Baked Ziti (page 139) or the Pad Thai (page 141). Add a green salad for a complete meal.

Serves 8

3 tablespoons olive oil

1 tablespoon Dijon mustard

1 tablespoon fresh lemon juice

½ teaspoon fresh lemon zest

1 teaspoon finely minced
   garlic

½ teaspoon salt

½ teaspoon black pepper

Dash of cayenne pepper

16 chicken wings, each halved at
   the joint with tip removed (just
   snip it off with kitchen shears
   or ask your butcher to do it)

1½ cups whole-wheat bread crumbs

1 cup freshly grated Parmesan
   cheese

6 tablespoons chopped fresh
   parsley

Dip Ingredients

1 cup fat-free yogurt

½ teaspoon chopped fresh
   parsley

½ teaspoon fresh lemon juice

¼ teaspoon fresh lemon zest

¼ teaspoon salt

¼ teaspoon black pepper

⅛ teaspoon Worcestershire sauce

1. Combine the olive oil, mustard, lemon juice, lemon zest, garlic, salt, pepper, and cayenne pepper in a small bowl and whisk together.

2. Place the chicken wings in a gallon-size resealable plastic bag and pour the marinade over them. Close the bag and marinate the wings in the refrigerator for 1 to 4 hours.

3. Preheat the oven to 425°F. Line a baking pan with foil and spray the foil with cooking spray. Set aside.

4. In a small bowl, combine the bread crumbs, Parmesan, and parsley. Dip each wing in the bread crumb mixture to coat and place it on the prepared pan. Bake on the lowest oven rack for 30 minutes, turning the wings over after 20 minutes.

5. While the wings are baking, combine all of the dip ingredients in a small bowl. Serve the wings warm with the dip.

~~~~~~~~ USE-WHAT-YOU-HAVE VARIATIONS ~~~~~~~~

Use any of these variations, or mix and match them according to your tastes.

VARIATION 1:   Instead of olive oil, try any other cooking oil.

VARIATION 2:   Instead of Dijon mustard, try any other mustard or barbecue sauce (preferably low-sugar).

VARIATION 3:   Instead of fresh lemon zest and juice (in wings and/or dip), try any other citrus zest and juice.

VARIATION 4:   Instead of garlic, try ½ teaspoon garlic powder or ½ teaspoon onion powder.

VARIATION 5:   Instead of cayenne pepper, try:

~ Any red pepper ~ A dash of any hot sauce ~ Chili powder.

VARIATION 6:   Instead of chicken wings, try:

~ 16 chicken breast strips, for a boneless version (cut 4 chicken breasts into 4 strips each) ~ 16 ounces extra-firm tofu, drained and cut into 32 strips or triangles ~ 16 ounces tempeh, cut into 32 strips.

VARIATION 7:   Instead of bread crumbs, try any breading, such as Panko (a type of flaky bread crumb from Japan), Matzo meal, or cracker crumbs.

VARIATION 8:   Instead of Parmesan, try any other highly flavored, hard grated cheese (such as Romano or Pecorino).

VARIATION 9:   Instead of fresh parsley (in wings and/or dip), try any other fresh leafy herb (like cilantro), half the amount of dried parsley, or any other dried herb.

VARIATION 10:   For the dip, instead of fat-free yogurt, try:

~ Any other plain yogurt (Greek, soy, etc.) ~ Reduced-fat sour cream (regular or nondairy).

VARIATION 11:   Instead of Worcestershire sauce, try:

~ Soy sauce ~ Tamari ~ Shoyu ~ Fish sauce ~ Steak sauce.

~ ~

Whole-Wheat Pasta with Mushrooms

This recipe first appeared in my column in *Health* magazine. It's a simple, flavorful dish. If you love mushrooms, you'll love this recipe. The truffle oil adds a complex level of mushroom-ness. I added it by accident and loved the result.

Serves 6

Pinch of garlic salt

12 ounces whole-wheat pasta
(any shape)

1½ tablespoons olive oil,
divided

1 shallot, sliced

1 package (3–5 ounces) sliced
shiitake mushrooms

1 package (3–5 ounces) sliced
mixed-mushroom blend

1 package (15–18 ounces) sliced
baby portobello mushrooms

1 teaspoon salt, divided

1 teaspoon black pepper,
divided

1½ tablespoons truffle oil

⅓ cup freshly grated Parmesan
cheese

2 tablespoons chopped fresh
parsley

1. Bring a large pot of water to a boil. Add the garlic salt to the water and cook the pasta according to the package directions.

2. Meanwhile, heat ½ tablespoon of the olive oil in a large nonstick pan on medium heat. Sauté the shallot. Add all of the mushrooms, turn the heat to medium-high, and cook for 5 to 6 minutes without stirring, or until browned on one side. Flip the mushrooms over and brown them on the opposite side for another 5 to 6 minutes. Season with ½ teaspoon of the salt and ¼ teaspoon of the pepper.

3. Drain the pasta. Toss the pasta in a large bowl with the mushroom mixture. Add the truffle oil, the remaining olive oil, and the remaining salt and pepper. Toss to combine. Top with the Parmesan and parsley. Serve hot.

~~~~~~~~ USE-WHAT-YOU-HAVE VARIATIONS ~~~~~~~~

Use any of these variations, or mix and match them according to your tastes.

VARIATION 1:   Instead of garlic salt, try any regular or seasoning salt.

VARIATION 2:   Instead of whole-wheat pasta, try any other pasta, preferably whole-grain.

VARIATION 3:   Instead of the shallot, try ¼ onion, chopped, any variety (including leeks and scallions).

VARIATION 4:   Instead of this recipe's exact mushroom mix, try any other mushroom or combination of mushrooms that you like.

VARIATION 5:   Instead of truffle oil, try any other good-quality, flavorful, cold-pressed oil.

VARIATION 6:   Instead of Parmesan, try any other hard grating cheese.

VARIATION 7:   Instead of fresh parsley, try any other fresh leafy herb, such as cilantro or basil.

~ ~

Lower-Fat Pasta Carbonara

I mentioned this recipe in Chapter 5 because I accidentally used vanilla soy milk instead of plain soy milk. *Not* good. Consider yourself warned. Use plain soy milk, not vanilla!

Serves 4

16 ounces whole-wheat
    spaghetti
¾ cup plain unflavored soy milk
2 whole eggs
½ cup freshly grated Parmesan
    cheese
1 teaspoon garlic salt, divided
1 teaspoon black pepper,
    divided

2 tablespoons butter (regular or
    nondairy)
8 slices organic turkey bacon,
    cooked until crispy and
    chopped
1½ teaspoons red pepper
    flakes

1. Cook the spaghetti according to the package directions. Meanwhile, in a large bowl, whisk together the soy milk, eggs, Parmesan, half the garlic salt, and half the pepper.

2. When the pasta is done, drain it and quickly put it directly into the bowl with the egg mixture. Toss to coat. The hot pasta will cook the eggs. When the pasta is coated with the egg mixture, mix in the butter, turkey bacon, red pepper flakes, and the remaining garlic salt and pepper. Serve immediately.

~~~~~~~~ USE-WHAT-YOU-HAVE VARIATIONS ~~~~~~~~

Use any of these variations, or mix and match them according to your tastes.

VARIATION 1:   Instead of whole-wheat spaghetti, try any other pasta, preferably whole-grain, in any shape you like.

VARIATION 2:   Instead of soy milk, try any other plain unflavored milk.

VARIATION 3:   Instead of Parmesan, try any other hard grating or shredded cheese.

VARIATION 4:   Instead of garlic salt, try any regular or seasoned salt.

VARIATION 5:   Instead of turkey bacon, try:
~ Prosciutto ~ Canadian bacon ~ Lean ham ~ Vegetarian bacon.

VARIATION 6:   Instead of or in addition to red pepper flakes, try chopped fresh parsley or peas.

~~~~~~

Lighter Chicken Pot Pie

Classic chicken pot pie is comfort food, but it's so heavy that it can make you feel like you want to die if you eat too much of it. This recipe takes the concept and lightens it up considerably. I talked about making this recipe in Chapter 5. It took a few tries to get it right. My *safety* in this recipe was to use Worcestershire sauce, which I think gives this pot pie that meaty, smoky zip.

Serves 6

1 pound boneless, skinless chicken breasts, boiled and shredded

2 cups mixed frozen peas and carrots

½ cup chopped celery

⅓ cup chopped onion

1⅓ cups chicken broth, divided

1 teaspoon garlic salt, divided

1 teaspoon black pepper, divided

⅔ cup oat flour

⅓ cup soy milk

2 teaspoons Worcestershire sauce

Premade double piecrust

1. Preheat the oven to 400°F. In a nonstick saucepan, combine the chicken, mixed vegetables, celery, and onion. Add 1 cup of the chicken broth and cook over medium heat until the frozen vegetables are tender, about 10 minutes. Taste and season with half the garlic salt and half the pepper.

2. In a separate saucepan over low heat, combine the oat flour and the remaining chicken broth and whisk it together until it thickens. Add the soy milk and whisk that in until it is smooth. Cook until the mixture begins to turn the color of peanut butter, about 5 minutes. Add the Worcestershire sauce and the remaining salt and pepper, then add this sauce to the chicken and vegetable mixture. Stir everything together until the sauce is well incorporated into the chicken and vegetables.

3. Put the bottom pastry crust in a pie pan. Pour in the chicken and vegetable mixture, then cover with the other pastry crust, pressing down the edges. Trim the edges so that they don't hang over the pie plate edge or they will burn. Make a few slits in the top for steam to escape. Bake for 35 minutes, or until the top crust is golden brown. Keep an eye on it as it bakes. If the edges are browning too quickly, put strips of foil over them. When the pie is done, let it stand for at least 20 minutes so that it can set. Cut into wedges and serve with a salad.

Use any of these variations, or mix and match them according to your tastes.

VARIATION 1:   Instead of boneless chicken breasts, try:
~ Removing the meat from a 2-pound purchased rotisserie chicken
~ Boneless, skinless turkey breast ~ Chopped precooked lean beef
(leftover) ~ Smoked tofu, cut into small cubes ~ Adding 1 cup additional
vegetables to make a vegetable pot pie.

VARIATION 2:   Instead of peas and carrots, try any other frozen mixed
vegetables.

VARIATION 3:   Instead of chicken broth, try any other broth or stock.

VARIATION 4:   Instead of onion, try 1 leek, chopped, white parts only or
2 shallots, thinly sliced.

VARIATION 5:   Instead of oat flour, try any other flour, preferably whole grain.

VARIATION 6:   Instead of garlic salt, try any regular or seasoned salt.

VARIATION 7:   Instead of soy milk, try any other plain unflavored milk.

VARIATION 8:   Instead of Worcestershire sauce, try:
~ Soy sauce (including tamari or shoyu) ~ Teriyaki sauce ~ ½ teaspoon
Liquid Smoke.

VARIATION 9:   Instead of a premade piecrust, try homemade piecrust.

~~~~~~

Vegetable Brown Rice

Sometimes you don't want dinner to be a big deal. You are a little bit hungry, but
you want something light and healthy. My answer: Vegetable Brown Rice with a

salad or a bowl of soup. If you are eating late, this is a good choice because you won't be weighed down digesting meat or dairy while you're trying to sleep. It's also really easy to make.

Serves 8 (leftovers make a good lunch)

2 cups raw brown rice

4 cups water

½ teaspoon garlic salt

½ cup chopped red bell pepper

½ cup frozen peas

2 tablespoons olive oil

½ teaspoon salt

½ teaspoon black pepper

¼ cup toasted sesame seeds for garnish (toast them in a dry nonstick skillet over medium heat, stirring constantly, just until they begin to turn golden brown)

1. Toast the rice by putting it in a large saucepan with no water. Warm over medium heat, stirring occasionally, until the rice releases a nutty aroma.

2. Add the water and garlic salt, then bring the rice to a boil. Reduce to a simmer. Add the red bell pepper, peas, olive oil, salt, and pepper.

3. Cover and cook until the rice is tender, about 45 minutes (taste it after about 30 minutes, then every 5 minutes). Serve warm sprinkled with the toasted sesame seeds.

~~~~~~~~~ USE-WHAT-YOU-HAVE VARIATIONS ~~~~~~~~~

Use any of these variations, or mix and match them according to your tastes.

VARIATION 1:   Instead of brown rice, try a different grain, but remember that grains vary in cooking time. Try:
~ Quinoa ~ Spelt ~ Bulgur wheat ~ Barley.

VARIATION 2:   Instead of garlic salt, try any regular or seasoned salt.

VARIATION 3:   Instead of red bell pepper, try any fresh chopped or frozen vegetables, such as any other color bell pepper, zucchini, summer squash, or artichoke heart.

VARIATION 4:   Instead of peas, try any fresh chopped or frozen vegetables, such as mixed frozen vegetables, green beans, corn, or asparagus (cut into 1-inch lengths).

VARIATION 5:   Instead of olive oil, try any other cooking oil or melted butter (regular or nondairy).

VARIATION 6:   Instead of sesame seeds, try any other seeds or chopped nuts.

~~~~~~

My Favorite Vegetable Recipes

I'm a big fan of vegetables, and if you are a Skinnygirl, I know you are, too. Vegetables are the Skinnygirl's secret weapon because they are nutrient dense, high in volume, and low in calories. Always add a great vegetable dish to dinner, if you can. You probably know what it's like to have your main course planned—you already have chicken or steak or salmon or something else in mind—but you need side dishes to fill in the meal. Vegetable dishes are the perfect solution. I know a lot of people still believe they don't like vegetables, but I can show you how to make vegetables that are so good, you'll want to cry. If you don't like vegetables, you just haven't had them cooked well. A vegetable cooked to bring out its full flavor is a beautiful thing. Try these recipes (and their variations) and you'll become a convert.

I'm not much of a steamed vegetable person. I think steamed vegetables taste pretty bland and boring. I prefer to roast or sauté them. Trust me, you aren't going to get fat because you cooked your vegetables in oil. The right herbs and spices make vegetables even more interesting. So, when you are looking for a side dish, consult the following recipes. I have a feeling that at least a few of them will win you over.

What to Do with Leftover Peas

What can I say? I had half a bag of frozen peas left over from creating another recipe the day I created this recipe. Simple and good. This recipe would work with just about any leftover vegetable you have in the refrigerator or freezer.

Serves 2 to 4

1 tablespoon olive oil
1 red onion, chopped into 1-inch
  pieces
½ teaspoon salt

½ teaspoon black pepper
2 cups leftover or frozen peas
1 clove garlic, minced

1. Heat a nonstick pan over medium heat. Add the olive oil, onions, salt, and pepper. Cook until the onions are soft and fully browned.

2. Add the peas and minced garlic. Cook until everything is heated through. Taste and add more salt and pepper if needed. Serve hot.

~~~~~~~~ USE-WHAT-YOU-HAVE VARIATIONS ~~~~~~~~

Use any of these variations, or mix and match them according to your tastes.

VARIATION 1:   Instead of olive oil, try any other cooking oil or butter (regular or nondairy).

VARIATION 2:   Instead of red onion, try:
  ~ Any other onion ~ 2 leeks, thinly sliced ~ 4 shallots, thinly sliced.

VARIATION 3:   Instead of peas, try any frozen vegetable, such as:
  ~ Green beans ~ Corn ~ Mixed vegetables.

VARIATION 4:   Instead of garlic, try ¼ teaspoon garlic powder or ¼ teaspoon onion powder.

~~~~~~

Easy Artichokes

If I'm going to make a fancy, complicated stuffed artichoke dish, then peeling fresh artichokes is worth the trouble. When I just want to eat artichokes without any fuss, however, I turn to this recipe. The trick is to cook the artichoke hearts until they are really crispy. Before you start making this recipe, defrost the artichokes in the refrigerator. Put them in there a day ahead. Before cooking, drain them very well in a colander for about 15 minutes and then press on them gently with paper towels

You could use the canned artichoke hearts (not the marinated kind), well drained, but they will be softer and will probably fall apart more easily. They probably won't actually get crispy, but they will still taste good, in a different way. If that's what you have, go ahead and try it.

Serves 2 to 4

1 tablespoon olive oil
1 package (about 9 ounces)
*   frozen artichoke hearts,*
*   defrosted and well drained*
½ teaspoon salt
½ teaspoon black pepper

1 teaspoon minced fresh
*   rosemary*
¼ teaspoon fresh lemon juice
3 tablespoons freshly grated
*   Parmesan cheese, divided*
1 teaspoon minced fresh parsley

1. Heat a nonstick pan over high heat. Add the olive oil, artichoke hearts, salt, and pepper. Cook without stirring until the artichokes are browned on one side, then toss. Continue to cook until the artichokes are crispy.

2. Add the rosemary, lemon juice, and 2 tablespoons of the Parmesan. Toss to coat. Put the artichokes in a serving bowl and sprinkle with the remaining 1 tablespoon of Parmesan and the parsley.

Use any of these variations, or mix and match them according to your tastes.

VARIATION 1:   Instead of olive oil, try any other cooking oil, or butter (regular or nondairy).

VARIATION 2:   Instead of artichoke hearts, try mushrooms.

VARIATION 3:   Instead of fresh rosemary, try ½ teaspoon dried rosemary, or any other fresh leafy herb.

VARIATION 4:   Instead of fresh lemon juice, try any other citrus juice.

VARIATION 5:   Instead of Parmesan, try any other hard grated cheese.

VARIATION 6:   Instead of parsley, try fresh cilantro, or fresh basil.

~~~~~~

Roasted Lemony Asparagus

Try this recipe in the spring when asparagus is in season. Roasting brings out the tender, sweet, mellow flavor of asparagus. Always cut off the bottom inch of the stalks before cooking, because that is the part that turns woody. Stores and farmers' markets typically sell asparagus in bunches, and this recipe works for any average-size bunch, which might be ten stalks or twenty, depending on thickness. Don't worry about exact amounts.

Serves 2 to 4

1 bunch asparagus (bottoms
    trimmed)
½ teaspoon salt
½ teaspoon black pepper
½ tablespoon fresh lemon juice
1 tablespoon olive oil

¼ cup freshly grated Parmesan
    cheese, divided
2 tablespoons chopped fresh
    parsley, divided
4 cloves garlic, smashed

1. Preheat the oven to 350°F. Spray a baking dish with cooking spray. Place the asparagus stalks in the dish, side by side, in a single layer. Sprinkle with the salt and pepper. Drizzle with the lemon juice and olive oil. Sprinkle with half the Parmesan and half the parsley. Top with the smashed garlic.

2. Roast the asparagus for 25 minutes. Remove the garlic cloves and discard.

3. Serve the asparagus sprinkled with the remaining Parmesan and parsley.

~~~~~~~~ USE-WHAT-YOU-HAVE VARIATIONS ~~~~~~~~

Use any of these variations, or mix and match them according to your tastes.

VARIATION 1:   Instead of asparagus, try white asparagus or green beans.

VARIATION 2:   Instead of fresh lemon juice, try any other citrus juice.

VARIATION 3:   Instead of olive oil, try any other cooking oil or melted butter (regular or nondairy).

VARIATION 4:   Instead of Parmesan, try any other hard grated cheese.

VARIATION 5:   Instead of fresh parsley, try any other fresh leafy herb.

~~~~~~

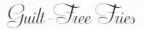

Guilt-Free Fries

Potatoes are a starchy vegetable, but they are still a nutrient-dense vegetable, so I'm including this seemingly decadent but actually good-investment recipe for fries. Skip the fast food and make these at home. You'll be glad you did.

Serves 4

4 baking potatoes

1 tablespoon olive oil

½ teaspoon salt

½ teaspoon black pepper

½ teaspoon paprika

1. Preheat the oven to 425°F. Cut the potatoes into wedges or strips, leaving the skins on. Toss them with the olive oil, salt, and pepper. Arrange them in a single layer on a foil-lined baking sheet. Sprinkle with the paprika.

2. Bake for 35 to 45 minutes, or until the potatoes are crisp. Serve hot.

~~~~~~~~ USE-WHAT-YOU-HAVE VARIATIONS ~~~~~~~~

Use any of these variations, or mix and match them according to your tastes.

VARIATION 1:   Instead of baking potatoes, try:

~ Fingerling potatoes, cut in half ~ Yukon Gold potatoes ~ Sweet potatoes or yams.

VARIATION 2:   Instead of olive oil, try any other cooking oil.

VARIATION 3:   Instead of salt, try any seasoning salt.

VARIATION 4:   Instead of paprika, try:

~ Garlic powder ~ Ground cumin ~ Chopped fresh herbs ~ Cinnamon (for sweet potato or yam option) ~ Any seasoning mix.

Chapter 10

Snacking Simplified

I used to have snacking anxiety. If I was hungry at 4 P.M. and knew I was going out for dinner, I would start to panic. What if I was "bad" and ate something? How could I justify that and eat dinner as well? If I did give in, the whole day, not to mention my mood, was ruined. The food noise would be deafening.

Discovering that snacking can aid in weight loss/maintenance was a revelation to me. Now I realize that if I'm hungry at four and I'm having dinner at eight, a snack is a really good investment because snacks decrease your appetite and stabilize your blood sugar. A snack is a minimeal that will keep you from going overboard later and attacking the bread basket, the dessert tray, and everything in between.

However, I don't believe in eating when you aren't hungry, just because the clock or a diet tells you to eat. You might not *need* to eat every three hours, or whatever some diet says. Snacking is also not an excuse to graze your way through the kitchen while you are cooking.

However, if you aren't going to eat for a few hours, don't freak out because you are hungry. Eat something. Have your good-investment snack, then do something else until it's time for dinner. Investing now saves you later. Remember, *your diet is like a bank account*. Snacks can help you keep it balanced.

If your kitchen is well stocked and organized, you should always be able to find a quick, easy, delicious snack when you need one. *Always*. Snacks are simple, but they shouldn't have to be boring or mindless. Make your snacks special *and* let go of the anxiety. Have a snack if you want one but don't schedule it. How will you know you are going to be hungry? At the end of the day, you will have eaten less if you go by your real hunger and snack according to your food voice.

Some people really do need to eat regularly because they don't notice they are starving until it's too late. If this is you, then *know thyself*. You know that you need to have a mid-morning, mid-afternoon, or evening snack to avoid getting into that situation. Snacking can keep you from bingeing, but it is also useful to keep you from simply overeating. For example, if you know you will be going to a party with a ton of great food, don't starve yourself. Have a snack first—something with protein—so that you can have your head on straight at the party and make better decisions.

Snacks can be as easy as toast with something on it, as fresh as a salad or a bowl of gazpacho, as comforting as warm grains with fresh herbs, as fun as flavored popcorn, or as sweet as a healthy cookie (consider any of the cookie recipes in this book) or my Faux Cheesecake from *Naturally Thin*. Here are some ideas. Let these inspire you to make your own creative snacks, and never go hungry again.

Whole-Grain Bruschetta with Tomatoes and Fresh Basil

Bruschetta is just toasted slices of bread with topping. It's an easy snack and a great way to use up a loaf of bread that is going stale. Bruschetta is easy to customize according to what you have. It's also good for parties because you can slice up a whole French baguette and make a tray full of bruschetta. For snacking purposes, just make two or three small slices and put something healthy on top. This is one good option, but see the many variations that follow. You can easily cut this recipe in half to serve one, or double it to serve four.

Serves 2

6 thin slices whole-grain
    French baguette or Italian
    bread
1 clove garlic
1 tablespoon plus 1 teaspoon
    olive oil

3 plum tomatoes, chopped
1 tablespoon fresh chopped
    basil
1 teaspoon balsamic vinegar
Salt and pepper to taste

1. Preheat the oven to 450°F. Arrange the bread slices on a baking sheet. Bake for 5 or 6 minutes, or until the bread looks lightly toasted.

2. Cut the garlic in half and rub the cut sides on each slice of bread. Drizzle the slices with 1 tablespoon of the olive oil.

3. Toss the tomatoes, basil, balsamic vinegar, and remaining olive oil together in a bowl. Divide this mixture between the bread slices, heaping it on top. Season with salt and pepper. Serve immediately.

Use any of these variations, or mix and match them according to your tastes.

VARIATION 1:   Instead of a French baguette, try your favorite bread, preferably whole-grain.

VARIATION 2:   Instead of this tomato-basil topping, try other toppings. Use your imagination. Here are some ideas:
~ Chopped olives with herbs or purchased tapenade sprinkled with fresh parsley ~ Chopped basil, pine nuts, and Parmesan, or purchased pesto sprinkled with a little feta ~ Olive oil, sun-dried tomatoes (rehydrated and chopped), and fresh basil ~ White beans with olive oil, basil, or arugula, salt, and pepper ~ Sautéed mushrooms with grated Parmesan or Pecorino, lightly drizzled with truffle oil ~ Fresh mozzarella slices with fresh tomato slices and chopped fresh herbs ~ Guacamole topped with fresh cilantro ~ Goat cheese topped with mixed greens, a drizzle of olive oil, and a sprinkle of lemon zest, salt, and pepper ~ Cream cheese and smoked salmon slices with chopped fresh dill or capers ~ Chicken salad with walnuts and grapes sprinkled with parsley ~ Tomato sauce and shredded mozzarella with dried oregano (broil or toast after topping).

Easy Beet Salad

This is a really quick salad when you want something fresh, sweet, and good for you. I love Melissa's trimmed, peeled, and steamed baby beets in a bag. They are all ready to go and have a great fresh-beet texture.

Serves 2

½ teaspoon salt

½ teaspoon black pepper

1 package (8 ounces) steamed
    beets, drained and cut into
    cubes

1 teaspoon apple cider vinegar

½ teaspoon fresh lemon juice

1 tablespoon crumbled goat
    cheese

1 tablespoon chopped fresh
    parsley

In a bowl, mix everything together except the goat cheese and parsley. Chill covered for 30 minutes or overnight, or enjoy immediately. Mix in the goat cheese and sprinkle the parsley on top just before serving.

~~~~~~~~ USE-WHAT-YOU-HAVE VARIATIONS ~~~~~~~~

Use any of these variations, or mix and match them according to your tastes.

VARIATION 1:   Instead of packaged beets, try roasted fresh beets: red, golden, or candy striped.

VARIATION 2:   Instead of apple cider vinegar, try any other vinegar.

VARIATION 3:   Instead of fresh lemon juice, try any other citrus juice.

VARIATION 4:   Instead of crumbled goat cheese, try any other flavorful, crumbled cheese.

~~~~~~

Classic Kettle Corn

Crunchy, salty, and sweet, kettle corn can satisfy a lot of different cravings. This recipe lets you relive the good old days when people made popcorn on the stove.

Serves 4

¼ cup raw sugar

¼ cup water

2 tablespoons vegetable oil

1 teaspoon salt

½ cup popcorn kernels (organic is best)

1. In a large nonstick pot over high heat, combine the raw sugar and water and stir until the sugar is dissolved. Add the vegetable oil and salt and stir to combine. Add the popcorn kernels and stir for 1 minute to distribute the oil–sugar mixture over the corn, then cover.

2. Once the popping starts, shake the pan well to distribute the kernels for even heating. Keep shaking. You can pick up the pan and give it a really good shake so it won't burn. When the popping gets wild, reduce the heat to medium. When the popping slows, remove from the heat and allow the last few kernels to pop.

3. Uncover and let cool for 5 minutes so that the sugar sets. Yum!

~~~~~~~~~ USE-WHAT-YOU-HAVE VARIATIONS ~~~~~~~~~

Use any of these variations, or mix and match them according to your tastes.

VARIATION 1: Instead of sugar, try:
~ Honey ~ Real maple syrup ~ Agave nectar ~ Flavored sugars, like vanilla or maple sugar.

VARIATION 2: For a savory version, replace the sugar with 1 tablespoon any seasoning salt, such as Cajun seasoning or Old Bay.

VARIATION 3: Instead of vegetable oil, try any other cooking oil.

~~~~~~

Bread Plus

Nothing irritates me more than the idea that bread is evil because it is made of "carbs," but it's just fine to gorge on bacon, cheeseburgers, steak, and eggs. A slice of bread with a good-investment topping is one of my very favorite quick snacks. It's a great way to satisfy your hunger and keep from getting ravenous later. Sometimes one of these half-sandwiches is all I need in the late afternoon and then I end up having a very light dinner.

It's not just about what you are eating when it comes to this kind of snack. It's about serving size. Remember, this is a snack—a slice of something with something on it. The options are endless. Here are some ideas based on some of the snacks I like to eat, but be creative and you'll discover your own favorites. My basic formula is one slice of bread, something with protein, some kind of vegetable or fruit, and some flavoring for interest:

- Nut butter: peanut, almond, cashew, sesame, with a small spread of fruit preserves or mashed banana.
- A slice of rice or soy cheese and a slice of fresh tomato.
- Tuna, chicken, egg, or tofu salad with lettuce and tomato.
- Lettuce, tomato, and turkey bacon with a light spread of mayon-

naise mixed with Dijon mustard and sprinkled with a little salt and pepper.

- Hummus with tomato and sprouts.
- A veggie burger with a slice of soy cheese, lettuce, tomato, and a sprinkle of salt and pepper.
- A fried or scrambled egg.

Chapter 11

Skinnygirl Drinks and Cocktails

'm referred to as a "fixologist" because I fix fattening cocktails, making them into cocktails that still taste great but have far fewer calories. Having a cocktail or two . . . or three . . . can add hundreds of calories to your day and only make you hungrier. I like to have a drink with friends, but I don't like the high sugar content of most of my favorite drinks. That's why I invented the Skinnygirl Margarita, which has become so popular that bartenders now know how to make them, and why I started my own line of Skinnygirl cocktails which you can now find in stores nationwide. (They are just 100 calories per serving, and the booze is in the bottle. The newest bottled flavors are the Skinnygirl Mojito and the Skinnygirl Cosmo. Find out more at skinnygirlcocktail.com.)

You can mix cocktails at home for a fraction of the calories. All you need to know is my Skinnygirl Fixologist Formula. If you learn nothing else from this book, this formula alone will make you glad that you bought it. You can apply this formula to *any mixed drink you like*. It will always work, and it's easy to memorize.

When I was in Turks and Caicos recently, they were serving a sweet rum punch drink. I just applied the formula and I drank it with everyone else, except that my version contained significantly fewer calories. Let's say it's Cinco de Mayo, and everybody is enjoying the frozen margarita mix. You want to participate, and you can. Just apply the formula. When I go out with friends, I explain the formula to the bartender—it takes just seconds—and I get a Skinnygirl version of whatever I'm in the mood to drink. It's easy, it's quick, and it works every time.

The Skinnygirl Fixologist Formula

Apply this four-step formula to any cocktail recipe and you'll be renovating that drink to be lighter with fewer calories and less of a morning-after impact.

1. Fill a rocks glass (short glass) with ice. Always use a lot of ice. As the ice melts, you can keep sipping the water.

2. Add clear liquor (pour while counting 1–2, or use a shot glass.) Clear liquor is cleaner and lighter with fewer impurities than dark liquor, so you are less likely to have a hangover (and the resulting desire to eat too much) the next day. I never drink dark liquor. Tequila and rum both come in clear versions. Gin and vodka are clear, and you can make vodka versions of just about any drink. I love tequila, but if the only kind available is brown, I'll have vodka.

3. Fill the glass the rest of the way up with club soda or seltzer, which should be another "classic" in your refrigerator. This reduces the strength of the drink and helps keep you hydrated.

4. Add just a splash of the sweet or fruity component that gives the drink its character—typically this will be a sweet liqueur, a sugary mix, or fruit juice. Go very light, with just enough flavor to accent the drink. Add fresh fruit for garnish whenever possible.

And that's it. It's so easy.

For that Cinco de Mayo party, ask for a clear tequila on the rocks with club soda and just a splash of that frozen machine mix everyone is drinking. Does the bartender look at you like you are crazy? Probably, but so what? You'll be glad you had that drink in the morning, when nobody else you went out with can button their jeans or open their eyes.

Maybe you are on vacation and you want a daiquiri or a piña colada, which is typically one of the most caloric drinks. A shot of rum, club soda, and a splash of daiquiri or piña colada mix tastes fantastic and perfect.

Maybe you are in New Orleans and you want to have a hurricane. Ask for a shot of clear rum over ice with club soda and just a splash of the hurricane mix. Try this anywhere.

This formula is just as easy to apply at home when you are mixing drinks for friends. If you have access to a cocktail book, it's fun to look for interesting drinks and then apply my formula. Or, check this list, find your favorite drink, and see how the Skinnygirl Fixologist Formula applies:

If you normally drink vodka and cranberry juice . . .	now you drink vodka and soda on the rocks with a splash of cranberry and a lime wedge
If you normally drink gin or vodka martinis . . .	now you drink gin or vodka and soda on the rocks with a splash of olive juice and an olive or a twist
If you normally drink margaritas . . .	now you drink clear tequila and soda on the rocks with a splash of citrus liqueur and 3 or 4 lime wedges
If you normally drink mojitos . . .	now you drink clear rum and soda on the rocks over crushed mint leaves with a dash of sugar or warmed honey or agave nectar and a lime wedge

If you normally drink rum and cola or diet cola . . .	now you drink clear rum and soda on the rocks with just a splash of cola or diet cola (add a lime wedge to make it a Skinnygirl Cuba Libre)
If you normally drink vodka Red Bulls . . .	now you drink vodka and soda on the rocks with just a splash of Red Bull
If you normally drink screwdrivers . . .	now you drink vodka and soda on the rocks with a splash of orange juice and an orange wedge

Also, when you are thinking about drinking, remember to apply the *Naturally Thin* concepts from my first book:

- Only drink clear liquor.
- Have a two-drink maximum. **On most occasions, stick to no more than two drinks. (I break this rule sometimes, but it's a good guideline to apply in general.)**
- Alternate a glass of water with every alcoholic drink. **Make this your personal unbreakable policy! (By the way, I break this rule all the time, but I do *try* to do this. Don't beat yourself up if you forget.)**
- Beware the wine refill. **Wine goes down too quickly, much more so than a mixed drink, especially when you are at a dinner party or a special event such as a wedding, and every time your wineglass is half finished, the server fills it up again. You can drink too much without realizing it. On a special occasion, I'll have a glass of wine or champagne, but I feel better the next day if I have a Skinnygirl cocktail instead. With a cocktail, you get one, you sip it, and you don't get more unless you decide to order another one, so you have a more conscious control over what you are drinking.**
- Eat protein and vegetables with alcoholic drinks rather than starch

and sugar. Balance your choices and consider an alcoholic drink the equivalent of dessert or bread. It all turns to sugar, so pick your poison. *You can have it all, but not all at once.* Notice how drinking makes you crave protein, not sweets, because alcohol is, effectively, a "sweet."

- Use the sugary mixes as flavoring only. I never say never, but most of the time, try to keep from having a whole glass of the sugary margarita mix from the machine or a drink that is mostly some other sugary component like cranberry juice or sour mix. If you do have one, take a few sips and treat it like a decadent dessert. Otherwise, it's so easy to make a Skinnygirl drink. Why do anything else?
- If you love dessert liqueurs, enjoy one over a lot of ice after dinner, *instead of* dessert. These are very sweet, so you only need a little. A dessert liqueur could replace one of your cocktail hour drinks or dessert, or just have some of it and a few bites of dessert. I'm not telling you what to do. I'm trying to help you see how to balance these choices so that you stay in control of what you are eating. I've been known to have a Sambuca on the rocks after dinner, but believe me, I always pay for it the next morning, especially if I've already been drinking other kinds of alcohol.

Building Your Home Bar

If you like to entertain and make drinks for friends at home, you'll love the Skinnygirl method of mixing because it's so fast and easy and you won't end up stuck behind the bar all night making complicated drinks. Having a well-stocked Skinnygirl home bar makes drink mixing even easier. You don't have to run out and get all these things at once, but if you gradually accumulate them, you can build a home bar that is functional and in keeping with *Naturally Thin* principles.

Tools

- Rocks glasses. These short glasses are handy for almost any drink. You can always serve drinks in taller glasses, but I rarely do, because a rocks glass doesn't hold as much, so you tend to drink less. The wide mouth makes sipping easier than in a tall, narrow glass.
- A small cutting board or bar board, for cutting citrus fruits.
- A sharp knife, for cutting lemon and lime wedges and peels.
- A shaker. Most bar tool sets have one. Shaking drinks is fun. You don't absolutely have to have a shaker, but if you want to buy one, take a look at skinnygirlcocktails.com or Bethenny.com for a link to my Skinnygirl bar accessories.
- A muddler. You can muddle cranberries, raspberries, mint, orange slices, or whatever you want to add to flavor your drink. (See "Muddle This" on page 172.) It's not absolutely necessary, but it's fun.
- A pitcher, for serving drinks to a group.
- A long-handled mixing spoon so that you can stir drinks when they are in the shaker or the pitcher. These also come in most bar tool sets.
- A corkscrew. Find one that you like and know how to use.

Liquor and Embellishments

I, of course, have every liquor ever made, including my newly released Skinnygirl Margarita premixed cocktail. But that's just me. I don't expect you to have a fully stocked home bar. If that's not your thing, just start with the basics:

- One or two bottles of your favorite clear liquor. This could include 100% agave clear tequila, good-quality clear rum, vodka (plain and/or flavored), or gin.
- One bottle citrus liqueur, such as Cointreau, Triple Sec, or Grand Marnier.

- One or two bottles of different liqueurs, for flavoring your favorite cocktails (such as Peach Schnapps, Midori, Limoncello, Elderflower, ginger, apple, etc.). Remember that you only need a little splash because these are mostly sugar. Choose your favorite.
- Garnishes: a few lemons, limes, oranges, a jar of cherries, a jar of olives, and fresh mint leaves (if you like to make mojitos or juleps).
- Juices for making your favorite drinks. You might include orange juice, pineapple juice, cranberry juice, or more exotic choices like lychee, peach, passion fruit, mango, or pomegranate. Have one or two around all the time, then buy others if you need them for a special cocktail. If you like piña coladas, add light coconut milk to your list.
- Honey or agave syrup for sweetening drinks—a lighter option than the simple syrup called for in so many cocktails. If you like your cocktails on the dry side, you can usually skip the sweetener.

MUDDLE THIS

Muddling is a bartending technique that means you bruise citrus peels, berries, or herbs (like mint leaves) so that they release their natural oils into the drink. You can buy a muddler, which looks like a tapered stick with a blunt end. Look for natural wooden ones. This is ideal for muddling mint for your mojito, but you can also use a long-handled metal or wooden spoon or a long pestle if you have a mortar and pestle. You could even use the handle end of a cooking spoon or wooden mallet. When a drink calls for muddling, put the ingredients to be muddled (such as mint leaves and sugar, lime wedge, or berries) into the bottom of a thick glass or cocktail shaker and smash them around with the muddler or spoon. Then add the rest of the drink ingredients and stir. For example: muddle over-ripe or frozen defrosted berries in the bottom of a rocks glass. Add ice, a shot of vodka, club soda, and a splash of chambord. Garnish with a lemon wedge.

- Raw sugar for garnishing glass rims. Flavored colored sugars are fun, too. You can buy them made for this purpose.
- A bottle of club soda or seltzer. Also keep tonic water or diet soda around if you like them. You can even use diet soda as a flavoring for club soda, just not as the main event. Diet sodas and energy drinks are not good investments, even sugar-free. Use just a little. The artificial sweetener may actually make you crave sweets.
- Plenty of ice.

Once you've got a stocked bar and the Skinnygirl Fixologist Formula under your belt, you can make just about any drink, but just to inspire you, here are a few of my favorites. *Note:* I am not including variations in this chapter because these drinks are all just versions of the Skinnygirl Fixologist Formula. Any changes result in new and different drinks, so I encourage you to take these as inspirations and then start mixing and matching your favorite flavors within the parameters of the formula. Also, not every drink follows the formula exactly because I was testing and adjusting to find the perfect tastes. I encourage you to do the same. The formula is a guide and a baseline for your cocktail creations, but it can be tweaked. Don't be afraid to experiment. Cheers!

Skinnygirl Mojito

Mojitos made with mixes have a lot of sugar. Request the Skinnygirl version, or make your own at home. (The Skinnygirl mojito is also in stores now, pre-mixed for you.) I created this for Daisy Fuentes in my column in *Health* magazine. It won't weigh you down or make you feel like you just drank your dessert.

½ fresh lime, cut into 6 wedges

2 tablespoons torn fresh mint
    leaves

1 cup ice

1½ tablespoons fresh lime juice

½ teaspoon honey, gently
    warmed (microwave for
    5 seconds)

2 ounces clear rum

4 ounces club soda

Fresh mint sprig and lime wedge
    for garnish

1. In a martini shaker, muddle the lime and mint with a pestle or long spoon until well bruised and fragrant. Add 1 cup of ice and the lime juice.

2. Combine the honey, rum, and club soda in a glass or small bowl. Stir gently to dissolve the honey. Add this combination to the muddle mixture. Stir until the mixture is well chilled. Strain into a rocks glass filled with ice. Garnish with the mint sprig and lime wedge.

Skinnygirl Black-Eyed Susan

The next few drinks are my Skinnygirl versions of the classic Triple Crown cocktails, which I created for the Triple Crown horse races: the Kentucky Derby, the Preakness, and the Belmont Stakes. I was an NBC correspondent for the Derby and did a special show with Kathie Lee and Hoda as part of the *Today* show. This drink in particular is the signature drink of the Preakness.

3 tablespoons white rum
3 tablespoons club soda
1 tablespoon any citrus liqueur
   (such as Triple Sec)

1 tablespoon pineapple juice
1 tablespoon orange juice
Lemon wedge or peel for
   garnish

Combine all of the ingredients except the garnish in a shaker full of ice and stir to blend. Strain into a rocks glass filled with ice. Garnish with the lemon wedge or peel.

Skinnygirl Gin Julep

I created this recipe for the Derby. The classic Derby drink is the mint julep, which is made with bourbon and a lot of sugar. This is my version made with gin.

Serves 1

4 tablespoons gin
4 tablespoons club soda
8 fresh mint leaves plus 1 sprig for garnish
2 teaspoons honey (heat in microwave for 10 seconds), but you could also
   use real maple syrup or even molasses to give this drink the darker color
   of a real mint julep
½ cup crushed ice (crush in a blender so that it's very fine)

Combine all of the ingredients except the garnish in a shaker full of ice and stir to blend. Strain into a rocks glass filled with ice. Garnish with the mint sprig.

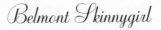

Belmont Skinnygirl

The Belmont Stakes is the third race in the Triple Crown.

Serves 1

4 tablespoons vodka
3 tablespoons club soda
1 tablespoon Peach Schnapps

1 tablespoon orange juice
Orange wedge for garnish

Combine all of the ingredients except the garnish in a shaker full of ice and stir to blend. Strain into a rocks glass filled with ice. Garnish with the orange wedge.

Skinnygirl Lychee Martini

I made lychee martinis for the girls on episode 4 of *The Real Housewives of NYC*, season 1, on Bravo. As often happens, I got a little too tipsy on these, so be careful. They are as delicious as they are exotic. You can buy canned lychees at the grocery store or Asian grocery.

Serves 1

2 ounces premium vodka
1 ounce lychee juice (from the
  can of lychees)

1 ounce club soda
2 lychees for garnish

Combine the vodka, lychee juice, and club soda in a cocktail shaker filled with ice. Shake well and strain into a chilled martini glass. Garnish with the lychees. *Optional:* Prior to making the drink, rim the glass with grated fresh ginger and dip in colored sugar (available in gourmet stores).

Skinnygirl Cosmo

Cosmos are such a popular drink, but I think they are too sweet. This version tastes delicious and has just a fraction of the sugar and calories. Indulge and fit into your jeans the next day.

Serves 1

2 ounces vodka
2 ounces club soda
Splash of cranberry juice

Juice from 2 lime wedges plus
1 lime wedge for garnish

Combine all of the ingredients except the garnish in a shaker full of ice. Stir and pour into a chilled martini glass. Garnish with the lime wedge.

Skinnygirl American "Virgin"

I created this drink for a Richard Branson Virgin America flight launch. You can make it a true virgin drink as is (no alcohol), or you can make it with peach vodka in place of the peach juice, for a less-than-virginal version.

Serves 1

2 ounces peach juice
2 ounces club soda
Splash of orange juice

Splash of lemonade
Lemon wedge for garnish

Combine all of the ingredients except the garnish in a shaker full of ice and stir to blend. Strain into a rocks glass filled with ice. Garnish with the lemon wedge.

Chapter 12

Skinnygirl Desserts to Die For

I'm immediately suspicious of any "diet" that says you can never eat sugar. I'm equally skeptical of anything "fat-free." Obviously, you should not eat a lot of sugar and fat, especially processed white sugar and trans fat, but desserts and sweets are part of life. To deny yourself completely will result in feelings of deprivation, bingeing, and rebellion.

I love dessert. When I do indulge, I don't gorge. I've learned how to have just a few perfect bites, savor them, then move on with my life. There are always those times when you have PMS or you are pregnant and you crave something sweet and it feels like a drug you need. That's part of life, but if you allow yourself the foods you love, you will never experience that panicky I-have-to-eat-it-all feeling. It's incredibly liberating.

Desserts are pretty bad investments if they are filled with sugar, flour, and fat. Or, you can renovate them, which is what this chapter is about. I've taken some desserts and lightened them up. At the same time, dessert has to be *worth the splurge,* so taste is my first priority. It can be yours, too, if you just remember one thing: Three's the charm.

Three's the Charm

When I renovate a dessert recipe, I take a regular recipe for something I want to make and then I do three things first, before I make any other changes:

1. I cut the fat in half.
2. I change the white sugar to raw sugar.
3. I change the white flour to oat flour.

These three small changes will barely impact the final result, and can even make it better, but require very little risk. Do just these three things to your favorite dessert recipe and know you are doing something good for yourself.

You can almost always cut the fat in a recipe at least in half and it will still work out fine. If the recipe says ½ cup of butter or oil, I'll experiment with ¼ cup. It doesn't always work, but more often than not, it's a success. You can substitute some or all of the oil for the same things you used to substitute for eggs: mashed bananas, butternut squash or pumpkin puree, applesauce, and prune puree. Most of the time, however, this isn't necessary.

Changing the white sugar to raw sugar adds nutrients that are stripped from processed sugar, and I think it has a more interesting taste. White sugar is highly processed. Natural sugars have the same calorie content, but they contain more nutrients. White sugar is stripped of everything, and some studies show that it can actually make you hungrier. Think about sweeteners in terms of the ideal ingredients scale. White sugar is on the not-ideal side. In the middle are less processed sugars like raw or turbinado sugar and Sucanat. A piece of sugar cane would be the ideal, but that's obviously not realistic. Honey and real maple syrup are in a more natural form, but they don't always work for baking. Remember my exploding muffins? Substituting natural liquid sweeteners like honey, maple syrup, or agave nectar for dry granulated sweeteners is a bigger risk because you are changing the proportions of liquid to dry ingredients, and that can skew your result. For frosting, natural liquid sweeteners work better, but sometimes I do use confectioners' sugar. They haven't made a natural version yet that I know of.

Finally, changing the white flour to oat flour (or any other whole-grain flour, like whole-wheat pastry flour) adds nutrients, a more complex flavor, and more fiber. Oat flour is my go-to flour. So many people avoid wheat that I just use oat flour by default, and I like its sweeter taste. It's also a better nutritional investment than white flour, which, like white sugar, is highly processed and stripped of most of its nutrients. Even though processing adds back nutrients, white flour is pretty far removed from its natural form.

By the way, whole-grain flour is a great choice for things like pizza dough and bread because it has a grainy, nutty taste, but its coarse grains aren't always appropriate for delicate desserts such as lemon cake or angel food cake. Instead, when I do use wheat flour, I like whole-wheat *pastry* flour, which contains the nutrients from whole-wheat flour but is milled into a finer texture so that it works much better in sweet baked goods.

These three changes are easy to do and easy to remember, and they can change the way you make dessert. You'll get to have your cake and eat it, too.

Skinnygirl Baking Tips

Besides your "three's the charm" rules, here are some other Skinnygirl baking strategies:

- Lose the eggs or some of the eggs. If I see a recipe that takes 4 eggs, I'll always try it with 2 eggs and 2 egg whites (2 egg whites equals 1 whole egg). It's taking a risk, but often you can't even tell the difference. You can also substitute a lot of different things for eggs in baking and leave them out completely. One large egg contains about 4 tablespoons or ¼ cup of fluid, so substitute an equivalent amount according to your recipe. Good substitutions include mashed bananas, butternut squash or pumpkin puree, applesauce, and prune puree (as in prune baby food). You could also try any yogurt. However, if you substitute out the eggs, your recipe might not turn out with the same texture or structure as the original, but that doesn't mean it won't be good. Also, egg substitute will not work for soufflés, meringues, flourless chocolate cake, or other recipes that are based on the structure of real eggs.

Before you decide on a good egg substitute, think about your substitution and how that flavor would fit into your recipe. For example, banana works well in a recipe with chocolate because these two strong flavors balance and complement each other. However, you wouldn't want to use bananas in something like a lemon tart because the banana would overpower the light, delicate flavor of the lemon. Applesauce might work better. Prune puree would work with chocolate recipes or in most cookies. It won't work in a sugar cookie because it's a dark color, so think about the color, too. Butternut squash or pumpkin puree tastes delicious in cinnamon-rich baked goods like spice cake, and carrot cake.

- Try nondairy butter and shortening. I like to use nondairy butter and shortening instead of regular butter and shortening because these don't have the saturated fat content of butter or the trans fat content of margarine. Better fats are better investments. Earth Balance brand is good.

- The darker the better. I like to use dark chocolate instead of milk chocolate. Dark chocolate has antioxidants that are really good for you. Milk chocolate is more sugary.

- Know your milk options. I don't usually like to drink regular milk so I normally use soy milk, but since my doctor suggested that I cut back on both dairy and soy, I've been exploring other milk options. I've discovered great alternatives to soy milk such as almond milk, rice milk, coconut milk, hemp milk, cashew milk, and oat milk. You can use any of these in place of regular milk when making desserts. You can also substitute low-fat or skim milk for regular milk or cream, and in baked goods, you can also try low-fat buttermilk, for a tangier taste. Each kind of "milk" will yield a slightly different taste, but they are all good. Flavored milks can add an interesting effect to baked goods, too. Try vanilla or even chocolate soy, rice, or almond milk if you want to pump up the flavor.

- Add antioxidants. Increase the antioxidant content in muffins, cookies, and cake by adding a few tablespoonfuls of beet juice, beet puree, or carrot juice. Also add fresh or dried fruit, such as blueberries, cherries, cranberries, and raisins, whenever you think it would make a nice addition.

How-Is-This-So-Moist Chocolate Cake with Peanut Butter Glaze

When I first made this recipe, my fiancé and I stared at each other for days afterward, marveling at how moist and delicious this cake was. We couldn't believe it. I even accused him of dumping a stick of butter into the batter when I was in the bathroom. I kept looking at the recipe trying to figure out what made it so moist. It really is the dessert mystery of all time, as far as I'm concerned.

This recipe is wheat-free, vegan, and *easy*. I make this cake in a loaf pan so that each slice has just a little bit of the delicious peanut butter glaze, but you could also make it in a round or square cake pan or a release pan, or you could make cupcakes. Just be sure to use plenty of cooking spray and parchment paper. Make this recipe for any special occasion or just because you want chocolate cake.

Serves 12

1 ¼ cups oat flour

1 cup raw sugar

⅓ cup unsweetened cocoa
    powder (the darker and
    higher quality, the better)

1 teaspoon baking soda

½ teaspoon salt

1 cup warm water

1 teaspoon real vanilla extract

2 tablespoons vegetable oil

1 teaspoon apple cider vinegar

1. Preheat the oven to 350°F. Put all of the ingredients in a bowl and stir until combined.

2. Pour the batter into a loaf pan coated with cooking spray. Bake 40 to 50 minutes, rotating the pan about halfway through the baking time. When a tooth-pick inserted into the middle comes out clean, it's done. However, I like my cake a little bit underdone and gooey. If some moist crumbs cling to your toothpick, you can consider that done.

3. Let the cake cool completely, then top with Peanut Butter Glaze (recipe follows). Slice and serve.

Peanut Butter Glaze

½ cup raw sugar

2 tablespoons canola oil

2 tablespoons soy milk

2 tablespoons creamy 100%
    peanut butter (the natural
    kind, no added sugar)

2 tablespoons unsweetened cocoa
    powder

2 teaspoons real vanilla extract

Combine all of the ingredients in a bowl and mix with a hand blender until the sugar crystals are dissolved. If they aren't dissolving, you can gently heat the mixture until they do (heat on low on the stove or on 50 percent power in the microwave, stirring every 20 seconds). Be careful of spattering when blending this recipe—I spattered this all over my kitchen blinds! Spread the glaze on the cake.

~~~~~~~~ USE-WHAT-YOU-HAVE VARIATIONS ~~~~~~~~

Use any of these variations, or mix and match them according to your tastes.

VARIATION 1: Instead of oat flour, try any other flour, preferably whole grain (especially whole-wheat pastry flour) but also spelt flour or gluten-free flour (like brown rice flour).

VARIATION 2: Instead of raw sugar, try any other granulated natural sweetener.

VARIATION 3: Instead of vanilla extract, try any other extract you think would taste good with chocolate and peanut butter (I might try almond or maple).

VARIATION 4: Instead of vegetable oil, try any other cooking oil or melted butter (regular or nondairy).

VARIATION 5: Instead of apple cider vinegar, try white vinegar.

VARIATION 6: For the glaze, instead of raw sugar, try ⅓ cup agave syrup or ⅓ cup real maple syrup.

VARIATION 7: Instead of canola oil, try any nonflavored oil, especially any mild cooking oil or nut oil.

VARIATION 8: Instead of soy milk, try any other plain or flavored milk.

VARIATION 9: To make a plain chocolate glaze, substitute melted nondairy or regular butter for the canola oil and leave out the peanut butter.

VARIATION 10: To make a peanut butter glaze without the chocolate, leave out the cocoa powder.

VARIATION 11: Instead of spreading the glaze on the cake, spread it on a plate and place the cake on top of the glaze.

VARIATION 12:   To make the glaze thicker and more like a frosting, refrigerate it
for at least 30 minutes.

VARIATION 13:   To make the glaze thinner and better for drizzling, add more
soy milk, 1 teaspoon at a time, until you get the consistency of syrup.

VARIATION 14:   Forget the glaze and top with fruit topping.

~~~~~~

Brownie Cookies

These cookies are perfect for when you need great chocolate flavor. They have
just a little fat from the nondairy butter, and bananas replace the eggs. When I
developed this recipe, it was my intention to make cookies, but Jason said they
tasted more like brownies. Bake this recipe in cookie form or in a pan, as actual
brownies.

Makes about 24 small or 12 large cookies

½ cup nondairy butter, softened

1½ cups raw sugar

½ banana, mashed

2 teaspoons real vanilla extract

2 cups oat flour

⅔ cup cocoa powder

¾ teaspoon baking soda

¼ teaspoon salt

2 cups semisweet chocolate chips

1. Preheat the oven to 350°F. In a large bowl, beat the butter, sugar, banana,
and vanilla extract with a hand mixer until light and fluffy.

2. In a separate bowl, combine the flour, cocoa powder, baking soda, and
salt. Stir the flour mixture into the butter mixture until well blended. Stir in the
chocolate chips. Drop by rounded teaspoonfuls onto ungreased baking sheets.

3. Bake for 8 to 10 minutes, or just until set. Cool slightly on the baking sheets
before transferring to wire racks to cool completely.

Use any of these variations, or mix and match them according to your tastes.

VARIATION 1:   Instead of nondairy butter, try:

~ Regular butter ~ Canola oil (the cookies will be thinner and spread out more) ~ Coconut oil ~ Trans-fat-free shortening.

VARIATION 2:   Instead of raw sugar, try any other granulated natural sweetener.

VARIATION 3:   Instead of mashed banana, try:

~ Butternut squash puree ~ Pumpkin puree ~ Banana puree (baby food) ~ Prune puree (baby food) ~ Applesauce.

VARIATION 4:   Instead of oat flour, try any other flour, preferably whole-grain, especially whole-wheat pastry flour.

VARIATION 5:   Instead of chocolate chips, try:

~ 2 cups mini–chocolate chips (for more chips in each cookie) ~ 1½ cups chocolate chips and ½ cup chopped nuts, such as walnuts, pecans, almonds, or peanuts ~ 1 cup chocolate chips and 1 cup raisins or any other dried fruit ~ 1 cup chopped dried fruit.

~~~~~~

Not-So-Red Velvet Cupcakes

Here's the deal with this recipe, which I wrote about earlier but want to reiterate here. Red velvet cake is a very red cake that is traditional in the South. It's basically just white cake with red food coloring and a little bit of cocoa. I don't like to use food coloring because it's artificial, so I had the idea that I would use beet juice from a can of beets to color the cake red while adding some nutrients. The batter turned a beautiful pink, but when I baked it, the color did not translate at all. This cake isn't going to win any beauty contests, but it was so good that I almost wept. I did a blind taste test between "real" red velvet cake and this recipe, and mine tasted the same as the cake with the food coloring, if not better.

This cake is so delicious, you won't believe it. However, it is very delicate, so that's why I made it into cupcakes with liners. You could make this recipe in two 8-inch-round cake pans, but be sure to line the pans with parchment paper and spray them well with cooking spray, then dust them with flour. Otherwise, the cakes will stick to the pans and fall apart. An even better idea is to use a release pan so that you don't have to turn out the cake onto a plate. Just release the sides and frost. The cupcakes freeze well, so you can frost them and put them in the freezer, then take one out whenever you need a cupcake fix.

Makes about 24 cupcakes

2½ cups oat flour

1½ cups raw sugar

1 teaspoon baking powder

1 teaspoon baking soda

1 teaspoon salt

1 teaspoon cocoa powder

¾ cup vegetable oil

1 cup low-fat buttermilk

2 large eggs, at room temperature

3 tablespoons beet juice (from a can of beets)

1 teaspoon white vinegar

1 teaspoon real vanilla extract

1. Preheat the oven to 350°F. Put liners in cupcake or muffin pans. If you don't have enough pans for 24 cupcakes, make this recipe in batches.

2. In a large bowl, sift together the flour, sugar, baking powder, baking soda, salt, and cocoa.

3. In a separate bowl, whisk together the vegetable oil, buttermilk, eggs, beet juice, vinegar, and vanilla extract.

4. Combine the flour and oil mixtures and beat with an electric mixer until the batter is very smooth, about 2 minutes. Pour the batter into the cupcake liners and bake for about 20 minutes, rotating the pan after 10 minutes.

5. After the cupcakes cool completely, frost them with Cream Cheese Frosting (recipe follows).

Cream Cheese Frosting

This frosting is so good that I would dip someone's foot in it and eat it. I've also been known to dip a spoon into it. It makes double what you will need for the cupcakes, so you can save half and enjoy it on something else later. Or, if you know you should definitely not have irresistible frosting in your refrigerator, just cut this recipe in half.

*8 ounces reduced-fat cream
  cheese, softened*
¼ cup nondairy butter, softened

½ teaspoon real vanilla extract
¼ teaspoon almond extract
1 cup confectioners' sugar

Mix all of the ingredients together in a large bowl and beat with an electric mixer until smooth. Refrigerate for at least 30 minutes if the frosting isn't firm enough. Frost cupcakes or any cake. Store leftover frosting in the refrigerator.

~~~~~~~~ USE-WHAT-YOU-HAVE VARIATIONS ~~~~~~~~

Use any of these variations, or mix and match them according to your tastes.

VARIATION 1: Instead of oat flour, try any other flour, preferably whole-grain, especially whole-wheat pastry flour.

VARIATION 2: Instead of raw sugar, try any other granulated natural sweetener.

VARIATION 3: Instead of vegetable oil, try any other cooking oil or melted butter (regular or nondairy).

VARIATION 4: Instead of buttermilk, try any plain yogurt or any other milk with 1 tablespoon vinegar or lemon juice stirred in—let it sit for a few minutes to sour.

VARIATION 5: Instead of eggs, try:
~ ½ cup beet puree (puree beets in blender) ~ ½ cup mashed banana or banana puree (baby food) ~ Ener-G egg substitute equivalent to

2 eggs (follow package directions) ~ ½ cup applesauce ~ ½ cup prune puree (baby food) ~ ½ cup soy yogurt.

VARIATION 7:   Instead of white vinegar, try apple cider vinegar.

VARIATION 8:   Instead of vanilla extract, try almond or raspberry extract.

VARIATION 9:   For the frosting, instead of cream cheese, try nondairy cream cheese.

VARIATION 10:   Instead of nondairy butter, try regular butter or coconut oil.

VARIATION 11:   Also try this cream cheese frosting on:
~ Carrot cake ~ Coconut cupcakes (top with shredded coconut) ~ Chocolate cupcakes ~ As a filling sandwiched between cookies. (These look nice arranged on a platter. To make Skinnygirl Whoopie Pies, sandwich this frosting between the Brownie Cookies in this chapter.)

~ ~

Boo Boo Banana Bread

My dog's name is Cookie, but her nickname is Boo Boo, so we thought it was the perfect name for this banana bread (although you shouldn't give it to your dog because it has chocolate in it). I created this recipe simply because I had three overripe bananas and wondered what to do with them. I looked up banana bread recipes, then started making adjustments. Overripe bananas are the best to use in baking because they are the sweetest. They can even be really brown. This banana bread is amazingly moist. It's great for breakfast or an afternoon snack. You won't believe how good it is.

Makes 1 loaf

1 cup raw sugar	*1 teaspoon real vanilla extract*
1 tablespoon butter (regular or nondairy)	*1 cup oat flour*
	¾ teaspoon baking powder
1 cup mashed overripe bananas (2 or 3 bananas)	*½ teaspoon baking soda*
	¼ teaspoon salt
1 egg	*½ cup semisweet chocolate chips*

1. Preheat the oven to 350°F. Combine all of the ingredients in a bowl and mix well.

2. Cut a piece of parchment paper to fit the bottom of a loaf pan. Put it in the bottom of the pan and spray it with cooking spray. Pour in the batter and cover it loosely with foil.

3. Bake for 30 minutes. Remove the foil, then bake for another 20 minutes, or until a toothpick inserted in the middle comes out *almost* clean (moist crumbs are fine). Cool completely, then slice and serve.

~~~~~~~~ USE-WHAT-YOU-HAVE VARIATIONS ~~~~~~~~

Use any of these variations, or mix and match them according to your tastes.

VARIATION 1:   Instead of raw sugar, try any other granulated natural sweetener.

VARIATION 2:   Instead of bananas, try:

~ Applesauce ~ Pumpkin puree ~ Butternut squash puree.

VARIATION 3:   Instead of the egg, try:

~ ¼ cup applesauce ~ ¼ cup prune puree (baby food) ~ ¼ cup soy yogurt.

VARIATION 4:   Instead of vanilla extract, try:

~ Almond extract ~ Coconut extract ~ Banana extract.

VARIATION 5:   Instead of oat flour, try any other flour, preferably whole-grain, especially whole-wheat pastry flour.

VARIATION 6:   Instead of chocolate chips, try:

~ Any chopped nuts ~ Dried pineapple ~ Dried blueberries ~ Shredded coconut.

~ ~

Oatmeal Raisin Cookies

These cookies are moist, delicious, and relatively virtuous in the cookie spectrum. You can vary this recipe in so many ways, replacing different dried fruits, nuts, or chocolate chips (or a combination) for the raisins and altering the extracts according to what flavors you think would match your additions. For example, maple extract might be delicious in an oatmeal raisin cookie, but you might prefer a lemon extract in a version with dried blueberries.

Makes about 24 small cookies

1½ cups oat flour

½ cup raw sugar

½ teaspoon baking powder

½ teaspoon baking soda

½ teaspoon salt

¾ cup rolled oats

½ cup applesauce

⅓ cup soy milk

1 teaspoon canola oil

1 teaspoon real vanilla extract

½ cup raisins

1. Preheat the oven to 350°F. In large bowl, sift together the flour, sugar, baking powder, baking soda, and salt. Add the oats, applesauce, soy milk, canola oil, and vanilla extract, stirring well, until everything is completely combined. Stir in the raisins.

2. Drop the batter by rounded teaspoonfuls onto ungreased baking sheets. Bake for 8 to 10 minutes, or just until set. Be careful not to overbake the cookies. They taste better when they are a little bit soft. Cool slightly on the baking sheets before transferring to wire racks to cool completely.

Use any of these variations, or mix and match them according to your tastes.

VARIATION 1:   Instead of oat flour, try any other flour, preferably whole-grain, especially whole-wheat pastry flour.

VARIATION 2:   Instead of raw sugar, try any other granulated natural sweetener.

VARIATION 3:   Instead of applesauce, try:
~ Butternut squash puree ~ Pumpkin puree ~ Prune puree (baby food) ~ Mashed bananas or banana puree (baby food).

VARIATION 4:   Instead of soy milk, try any other plain or flavored milk.

VARIATION 5:   Instead of canola oil, try any other cooking oil or melted butter (regular or nondairy).

VARIATION 6:   Instead of vanilla extract, try any other extract you think would fit the recipe.

VARIATION 7:   Instead of raisins, try:
~ Any other dried fruit that you think would match the extract you want to use ~ Mini–chocolate chips ~ Any chopped nut ~ Shredded coconut.

~~~~~~

Joyful Heart Chocolate Chip Cupcakes

In my first book, *Naturally Thin,* I included a recipe for Joyful Heart Muffins. They are low-fat, wheat-free, and dairy-free. Since then, I've made another version of that recipe, switching the chocolate chips to mini–chocolate chips, slightly increasing the amount of the chips, and frosting the cupcakes with chocolate frosting. *Voila,* a breakfast muffin is transformed into a cupcake. I hope you'll try this. It's one of my favorites.

Makes 8 cupcakes

1 cup unsweetened applesauce
½ cup raw sugar
1 teaspoon real vanilla extract
1 teaspoon almond extract
1 teaspoon canola oil
¾ cup oat flour

⅓ cup unsweetened cocoa powder
2 teaspoons baking powder
½ teaspoon baking soda
½ teaspoon salt
Pinch of cinnamon
⅔ cup mini–chocolate chips

1. Preheat the oven to 375°F. Spray a muffin or cupcake tin with cooking spray or put liners into a muffin or cupcake tin to make 8 cupcakes.

2. In a small bowl, combine the applesauce, sugar, vanilla extract, almond extract, and canola oil. Stir and set aside to allow the sugar crystals to dissolve.

3. In a large bowl, sift together the oat flour, cocoa powder, baking powder, baking soda, salt, and cinnamon. Add the applesauce mixture and stir until everything is combined. Fold in the mini–chocolate chips.

4. Using a 3-ounce ice-cream scoop or large spoon, portion the batter into the tin to make 8 cupcakes. Bake for 20 minutes, or until the tops are firm to the touch.

5. Cool completely, remove from the tin, and frost with Chocolate Frosting (recipe follows).

Chocolate Frosting

1 cup nondairy butter
4 cups confectioners' sugar
2 tablespoons real vanilla
  extract

4 tablespoons soy milk
½ cup cocoa powder
Pinch of salt

Mix all of the ingredients together in a large bowl and beat with an electric mixer until very smooth. If the frosting is too thick, add a little more soy milk. If it is too thin, refrigerate for 30 minutes. Frost cupcakes or any cake. Store leftover frosting in the refrigerator.

Use any of these variations, or mix and match them according to your tastes.

VARIATION 1:   Instead of applesauce, try:
~ Butternut squash puree ~ Pumpkin puree ~ Prune puree (baby food) ~
Mashed bananas or banana puree (baby food).

VARIATION 2:   Instead of raw sugar, try any other granulated natural sweetener.

VARIATION 3:   Instead of the vanilla and almond extract combination, try:
~ Leaving out the almond extract and doubling the amount of vanilla
extract ~ Leaving out the vanilla extract and doubling the amount of
almond extract ~ Replacing either extract for a different extract, such as
orange, coconut, or raspberry.

VARIATION 4:   Instead of canola oil, try any other cooking oil or melted butter
(regular or nondairy).

VARIATION 5:   Instead of oat flour, try any other flour, preferably whole-grain,
especially whole-wheat pastry flour.

VARIATION 6:   Instead of cocoa powder, try leaving it out and increasing the
flour by 1/3 cup.

VARIATION 7:   Instead of cinnamon, try leaving it out.

VARIATION 8:   Instead of mini–chocolate chips, try:
~ Any chopped nuts ~ Dried cherries ~ Dried cranberries ~ Peanut
butter chips ~ White chocolate chips ~ Shredded coconut.

VARIATION 9:   For the frosting, instead of nondairy butter, try regular unsalted
butter or coconut oil.

VARIATION 10:   Instead of soy milk, try any other plain or flavored milk.

VARIATION 11:   Also try this chocolate frosting on:
~ White cake ~ Yellow cake ~ Spice cake ~ Coconut cupcakes (top with
shredded coconut) ~ As a filling sandwiched between cookies.

~~~~~~

Ricotta Cheesecake

Whenever I fly on Delta Airlines, I look forward to those crispy Biscoff cookies they give you. On a recent flight, I told the flight attendant how much I liked them, and she gave me a bunch of packets. I used them in the crust for this recipe, but if you don't have those, you could use vanilla wafers or graham crackers or even chocolate chip or cinnamon Teddy Grahams, if you have little kids and always have these around. This is an excellent holiday dessert and has a lot less fat than traditional cheesecake. Incidentally, this is the recipe I made on the same day I made that horrible Latte Carbonara. The vanilla soy milk was a happy accident here. It was the first time Jason and I ever cooked together.

Serves 12

1½ cups plus 2 tablespoons ground-up cookies (put them in a plastic resealable bag and pound on them or put them in the food processor and pulse until they are crumbs)
2 tablespoons melted butter (regular or nondairy)

2 tablespoons apple juice
8 ounces part-skim ricotta cheese
8 ounces reduced-fat cream cheese
⅓ cup raw sugar
2 tablespoons vanilla soy milk
1 teaspoon real vanilla extract
2 eggs

1. Preheat the oven to 350°F. Combine the cookie crumbs, butter, and apple juice in a bowl. Spray a springform pan with cooking spray and cover the outside tightly with foil (you are going to put it in water and you don't want the water to leak into the cheesecake). Pat the cookie mixture into the bottom of the pan and press down on it so that it is flat and evenly distributed.

2. In a large bowl, combine the ricotta, cream cheese, sugar, milk, and vanilla extract with an electric mixer. Beat in the eggs until they are fully incorporated. Pour the batter into the prepared crust.

3. Put the cake pan into a larger baking or roasting pan and put the whole thing into the oven. Carefully pour water into the baking pan so that it surrounds the cheesecake pan in a water bath about 1 inch deep. Be careful not to get water into the cheesecake. This step might seem complicated, but it will keep your cheesecake moist.

4. Close the oven and let the cake bake for 60 to 75 minutes. Start checking on it after 50 minutes. When the edges of the cheesecake are just beginning to turn golden brown and a toothpick inserted into the middle comes out mostly (but not completely) clean, the cake is done.

5. *Very carefully* remove the cake from the oven so that you don't spill hot water on yourself. Let the cake cool completely, then refrigerate for at least 2 hours or overnight. Serve with the Fruit Topping (recipe follows).

Fruit Topping

This topping adds nutrients and delicious juicy fruit flavor to the cheesecake.

2 cups cherries, pitted and sliced
¾ cup water
1 tablespoon plus 1 teaspoon
 cornstarch
1 tablespoon plus 1 teaspoon
 raw sugar
½ cup apple juice

Mix all of the ingredients together in a small nonstick pan and heat over medium-low until the topping begins to thicken slightly. Serve over the cheesecake before cutting, or put a spoonful on each slice.

~~~~~~~~ USE-WHAT-YOU-HAVE VARIATIONS ~~~~~~~~

Use any of these variations, or mix and match them according to your tastes.

VARIATION 1: Use any sweet, crispy cookies or crackers for the crust, including:
 ~ Vanilla wafers ~ Gingersnaps ~ Graham crackers ~ Almond crisps ~
 Chocolate crisps ~ Oreos ~ Fortune cookies.

VARIATION 2: Instead of apple juice, try:
 ~ Orange juice ~ White grape juice ~ Cranberry juice.

VARIATION 3:   Instead of ricotta, try whipped cottage cheese or silken tofu.

VARIATION 4:   Instead of reduced-fat cream cheese, try nondairy cream cheese.

VARIATION 5:   Instead of raw sugar, try any other granulated natural sweetener.

VARIATION 6:   Instead of vanilla soy milk, try any other plain or flavored milk.

VARIATION 7:   For the fruit topping, instead of cherries, try:
~ Any fresh or frozen berries ~ Fresh or frozen chopped orchard fruit, such as peaches, nectarines, or plums ~ Any combination of fresh or frozen fruit pureed or not.

VARIATION 8:   Instead of raw sugar, try any other dry or liquid natural sweetener.

Part Three

Skinnygirl Special Features

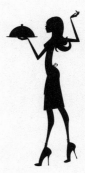

Chapter 13

Lightened-Up Holidays and Special Occasions

The holidays shouldn't be stressful, at least where cooking is concerned. (I can't do anything about visiting relatives.) You can make impressive meals for your holiday guests without spending the whole day in the kitchen. I hate babysitting food all day. I want to prepare a dish, put it in the oven, and set the timer. That's what this chapter is about.

The key to making a big meal with many elements is to prepare ahead. Assemble lasagna and refrigerate it. Make side dishes in advance and keep them covered in the refrigerator, then warm them up in the oven, in the microwave, or with a quick sauté on the stove.

I also advocate letting other people help. Why should you make everything? Desserts in particular are perfect for other people to bring. I like baking, but not when I'm also making an entire meal. Don't make yourself crazy baking a bunch of pies on Thanksgiving. Let your friends and family bring them, then doctor them with whipped cream, shaved chocolate, fresh fruit, or whatever you think would be appropriate. Another way to keep holidays simple is to make just a few dishes, then fill in the rest of the menu with easy no-cook foods.

Appetizers

Stimulate appetites and put people in the mood to celebrate with delicious and beautiful appetizers that won't spoil everyone's appetite for dinner.

- A platter of crudités such as carrots, broccoli, cauliflower, and asparagus, and a dip such as hummus, baba ghanoush, pesto, tapenade, or a mixture of half low-fat ranch dressing and half vinaigrette or any of the creamy dips from Chapter 14.
- An antipasti platter including bowls of marinated vegetables such as cherry peppers, artichoke hearts, olives, roasted red peppers, sun-dried tomatoes, baby pickles, and hearts of palm; slices of fresh mozzarella; dried meats such as prosciutto, pepperoni, and bresaola; and thin slices of baguette.
- Wooden cutting boards (IKEA has inexpensive ones) with different cheeses. Be sure to label them. IKEA sells placecards with holders for labeling cheese or make your own out of wire. You might include baby mozzarella, feta, brie en croute (brie cheese baked in pastry), and one or two other cheeses you like, such as Havarti, smoked Gouda, white cheddar, or flavored goat cheese. Add grapes, pears, or apples, and bread slices or good-quality whole-grain crackers.

WHO'S BLANCH?

Keep your vegetables bright and crisp with an expert trick. Prepare a large bowl of ice water and a large pot of boiling water. Put your vegetables, one kind at a time (e.g., all the carrots, then all the broccoli, etc.), into a heat-proof colander or strainer with a handle. Dunk them into the boiling water for about ten seconds (this is called blanching), then immediately plunge them into the ice water bath to stop the cooking immediately. This will bring out the bright color but retain the crisp texture. Now your crudités are ready to serve.

- A few different kinds of fancy snacks such as honey-roasted sesame cashews, wasabi peas, spiced pecans, and Marcona almonds.
- A selection of dips such as baba ghanoush, hummus, tapenade, or any of the dips in Chapter 14.

Side Dishes

For an easy holiday meal, spend your time preparing a few more time-consuming dishes, then round out the meal with easy side dishes that come together in minutes. Here are some ideas.

- Cranberry sauce: Cook 1 bag of fresh or frozen cranberries (½ pound) with 1 cup of water and 1 cup of sugar over medium heat until the mixture bubbles and the cranberries pop. Remove from the heat, stir in ¼ teaspoon each ground ginger, cinnamon, and orange peel, and refrigerate. You could also spoon this homemade cranberry sauce over goat cheese with whole-grain crackers for an appetizer.
- Roasted vegetables with salt, pepper, and a little lemon juice.
- Sweet potato puree, defrosted frozen butternut squash puree, or baked sweet potatoes. Heat and season with cinnamon, real maple syrup, or brown sugar, butter, and a little salt.
- Bread with homemade flavored butters. Divide a stick of butter between three or four bowls and let it soften at room temperature, then mix different ingredients into each: tapenade or chopped olives with olive bread, pesto with sourdough, chopped sun-dried tomatoes with whole-grain, or anything else that inspires you. Serve in ramekins. Flavored butters are elegant and impressive, even though they take just seconds to prepare.

Finally, have a tray of easy but impressive desserts, such as:

- Crushed fruit in red wine glasses tossed with almond extract, sugar, and lemon juice and topped with whipped cream.

- A platter of cookies or ice-cream cookie sandwiches made with low-fat ice cream or frosting.
- A platter of brownies or petit fours.
- Rainbow Fruit Skewers (from *Naturally Thin*).

Decorating

Decorating for the holidays makes the event seem even more special. Hang lights, make a simple centerpiece, place candles on the table and around the dining room, display food at different heights, and play appropriate music. Replace regular lightbulbs with rose-colored bulbs. Frame printed cocktail and dinner menus or write the menu on a stand-up chalkboard, especially for an Italian theme, as with the lasagnas in this chapter. These extra touches can add a big wow factor (for more ideas, see Chapter 14). Because it's not *all* about the food.

Holiday Menus

Let's start with a menu that's quick and easy. It can work for any holiday, or just for when you have a lot of people coming over for dinner. Add a special cocktail from Chapter 11 or any dessert from Chapter 12 to round out the event.

Lasagna Duo with Easy Dinner Salad

When having family, friends, or clients over for a holiday meal or just for a social event, the Lasagna Duo is very impressive, satisfying the carnivore and the vegetarian. You can make both lasagnas at the same time, so it doesn't feel like any extra work. There is minimal cleanup, allowing time for socializing.

Remember not to get too hung up on the recipe. If you can only find containers of ricotta cheese that are 16 ounces each instead of 15 ounces, or a big 32-ounce container, that's fine. A little variation won't make a noticeable difference.

You can bake these lasagnas at the same time, but you will probably have to increase the cooking time to about 45 minutes or even 1 hour because the oven will be doing twice the work. When the lasagnas are bubbling and look golden brown on the top, you will know they are ready.

Classic Lasagna

Serves 4

8 ounces whole-wheat lasagna
   noodles
1 pound turkey sausage, casing
   removed
16 ounces tomato sauce (don't
   be a hero—just buy the kind
   in a jar)
½ cup chopped fresh parsley
2 tablespoons chopped fresh basil

15 ounces part-skim ricotta
   cheese
1 teaspoon salt
1 teaspoon black pepper
4 ounces shredded part-skim
   mozzarella cheese
⅓ cup freshly grated Parmesan
   cheese

1. Preheat the oven to 350°F. Cook the lasagna noodles according to the package directions (or use no-boil noodles). Set aside.

2. In a nonstick skillet lightly coated with cooking spray, brown the turkey sausage. Stir in the tomato sauce. Set aside.

3. In a bowl, combine the parsley, basil, ricotta, salt, and pepper. Set aside.

4. Spray an 11½ × 7-inch baking pan with cooking spray (or any other pan that fits the lasagna noodles you have—this was the size that my recipe tester used). Ladle about one-third of the tomato sauce–meat mixture into the bottom of the pan. Cover with half the noodles. Spread half the herb–ricotta mixture over the noodles. Cover with all the mozzarella. Repeat with another one-third of the sauce, the remaining noodles, the remaining herb–ricotta mixture, then cover the whole thing with the remaining sauce. Sprinkle the Parmesan over the top.

5. Bake for 25 to 30 minutes, or until heated through and bubbling. Let sit for 15 minutes before cutting and serving.

~~~~~~~~ USE-WHAT-YOU-HAVE VARIATIONS ~~~~~~~~

Use any of these variations, or mix and match them according to your tastes.

VARIATION 1:   Instead of whole-wheat lasagna noodles, try no-boil lasagna noodles or gluten-free lasagna noodles.

VARIATION 2:   Instead of turkey sausage, try:
~ Any other lean sausage or ground meat ~ Veggie crumbles.

VARIATION 3:   Instead of tomato sauce, try jarred pasta sauce or canned tomatoes pureed in a blender and seasoned with salt, pepper, and herbs like basil and oregano.

VARIATION 4:   Instead of fresh parsley, try any other fresh leafy herb.

VARIATION 5:   Instead of fresh basil, try any other fresh leafy herb.

VARIATION 6:   Instead of ricotta, try part-skim cottage cheese, whipped or not or silken tofu.

VARIATION 7:   Instead of mozzarella, try any other mild shredded white cheese.

VARIATION 8:   Instead of Parmesan, try any other hard grating cheese.

~~~~~~

Pesto Vegetarian Lasagna

Serves 4

8 ounces whole-wheat lasagna
   noodles
15 ounces part-skim ricotta cheese
⅓ cup chopped fresh basil
¼ cup toasted pine nuts (toast
   gently in a dry skillet until
   golden)

⅓ cup packaged pesto
4 ounces shredded part-skim
   mozzarella cheese

1. Preheat the oven to 350°F. Cook the lasagna noodles according to the package directions (or use no-boil noodles). Set aside.

2. In a bowl combine the ricotta, basil, and pine nuts. Set aside.

3. Spray an 11½ × 7-inch baking pan with cooking spray (or any other pan that fits the lasagna noodles you have—this was the size that my recipe tester used). Spread one-third of the pesto in the bottom of the pan. Cover with half the noodles. Spread half the herb–ricotta mixture over the noodles. Repeat with another one-third of the pesto, the remaining noodles, the remaining herb–ricotta mixture, then cover the whole thing with the remaining pesto. Sprinkle the mozzarella over the top.

4. Bake for 30 minutes, or until heated through and bubbling. Let sit for about 15 minutes before cutting and serving.

~~~~~~~~ USE-WHAT-YOU-HAVE VARIATIONS ~~~~~~~~

Use any of these variations, or mix and match them according to your tastes.

VARIATION 1: Instead of whole-wheat lasagna noodles, try no-boil lasagna noodles or gluten-free lasagna noodles.

VARIATION 2: Instead of ricotta, try part-skim cottage cheese, whipped or not, or silken-tofu.

VARIATION 3:   Instead of basil, try any other fresh leafy herb.

VARIATION 4:   Instead of pine nuts, try chopped walnuts.

VARIATION 5:   Instead of pesto, try Homemade Pesto (see following recipe) or
sun-dried tomato pesto or any other flavor of purchased pesto.

VARIATION 6:   Instead of mozzarella, try:
~ Low-fat Monterey Jack ~ Provolone ~ Nondairy mozzarella ~ Leaving
it out.

~ ~

HOMEMADE PESTO

Doesn't it annoy you to buy a bunch of fresh herbs, use a handful, and watch the rest of them rot? So use them. One of the easiest ways is to make homemade pesto. You *could* buy premade pesto, and sometimes it's quicker, but really, this is so easy and freezes well, too. Pesto consists of five basic components: fresh basil, grated Parmesan, olive oil, pine nuts, and garlic, plus salt and pepper to taste. Put it all in the food processor or blender or use your immersion blender and blend until smooth. You can substitute other herbs or leafy greens, other hard grated cheese, and other nuts, too. For example, you could make pesto out of baby spinach, Pecorino, and walnuts. Here are the proportions:

- 2 cups fresh basil or other leafy herb or green
- ¼ cup grated Parmesan or other similar cheese (such as Asiago—or you can leave out the cheese and add more nuts)
- ⅓ cup extra-virgin olive oil or other oil
- ⅓ cup pine nuts or other nuts (such as walnuts)
- 3 cloves garlic, minced
- Salt and pepper to taste

Easy Dinner Salad with Simple Dressing

This easy salad goes well with both the Classic Lasagna and the Pesto Vegetarian Lasagna. If you chop your nuts finely and crumble the cheese into very small bits, a little will go a long way and every bite will have the fun stuff.

Serves 8

10 cups baby spinach

2 tablespoons finely chopped walnuts

4 tablespoons crumbled blue cheese

Salt and pepper to taste

In a bowl, toss the spinach, walnuts, and blue cheese together, season with salt and pepper, and drizzle with Simple Dressing (see the following recipe).

Simple Dressing

1½ tablespoons balsamic vinegar

1 tablespoon extra-virgin olive oil

1 teaspoon Dijon mustard

½ teaspoon salt

½ teaspoon black pepper

In a bowl, whisk all of the ingredients together and drizzle over salad. Toss to coat.

~~~~~~~~ USE-WHAT-YOU-HAVE VARIATIONS ~~~~~~~~

Use any of these variations, or mix and match them according to your tastes.

VARIATION 1:   Instead of baby spinach, try any other leafy salad greens.

VARIATION 2:   Instead of walnuts, try any other chopped nuts.

VARIATION 3:   Instead of blue cheese, try any other crumbled or shredded cheese.

VARIATION 4:   In the dressing, instead of balsamic vinegar, try any other vinegar or citrus juice.

VARIATION 5:   Instead of extra-virgin olive oil, try any other good-quality cold-pressed oil.

VARIATION 6:   Instead of Dijon mustard, try any other plain or flavored mustard.

~~~~~~

Holiday Dinner for 12

Whether it's Thanksgiving, Christmas, Easter, or whatever, this traditional menu of Roast Turkey, Sweet Potato Soufflé, Wild Rice, Low-Fat Corn Pudding, Green Bean Casserole, and Ricotta Cheesecake (page 195) will make everybody feel very comfortable and cozy. These recipes are so easy to make because you do almost everything ahead of time. One to three days before your event, make the mashed sweet potatoes for the Sweet Potato Soufflé. Also make the Wild Rice, Low-Fat Corn Pudding, and Green Bean Casserole. Put everything in the refrigerator, sealed. One or two days before the meal, make the cheesecake and refrigerate it as well.

On the day of your event, all you have to do is get the turkey in the oven. Then you can relax and enjoy the holiday. When you take the turkey out, it needs to sit for about 30 minutes. Leave the oven on and put the Wild Rice, Low-Fat Corn Pudding, and Green Bean Casserole in to warm up. Whip the egg whites and assemble the Sweet Potato Soufflé, then let it bake while you are putting everything else on the table. Slice the turkey and you're ready for dinner. You'll have all this amazing food and you won't be stressed at all.

Remember, whenever possible, to purchase premade ingredients and ask people to bring things. Especially during the holidays, you do not need to be a hero!

Roast Turkey

Making a turkey isn't exactly easy. It's time-consuming, but the result is so impressive that you might decide the effort is worth it, at least once a year. I'm not going to lie to you—roasting a turkey takes some work. The bottom line is that you are not going to leave the house while that turkey is in the oven. Name your turkey Howard or Larry or whatever, because you are going to be in a relationship with him, and that relationship is going to take some time.

Everybody has a different opinion about what to put on or in a turkey. In general, you are going to lube him up, salt and pepper him, and then baste him until you can't stand to baste him anymore. You need to watch that turkey, because if he gets too brown, you need to cover him with a foil blanket. If he isn't crispy enough, you need to uncover him and baste him some more. Start basting even before the turkey has released any juice into the pan. This is why I include putting some chicken broth on the stove while the turkey is roasting. Use that to baste (better than basting with oil), and then when the turkey gets going, baste with the turkey's own juices. Frequent basting—even every 15 minutes or so—makes a big difference in the result.

When the relationship is over, if you did your part, he'll reward you with a fabulous holiday meal. If you are commitment-phobic, just buy and roast a turkey breast. It's much faster.

Serves 12

1 turkey, approximately 16 to
    18 pounds, or 1 turkey breast
    if you prefer to serve white
    meat only (note shorter
    cooking time)
1 cup white wine
1 onion, cut into fourths, for
    giblet broth

1 carrot, cut into large pieces,
    for giblet broth
1 tablespoon chopped fresh sage
2 tablespoons chopped fresh
    thyme
1 bay leaf
1 teaspoon salt plus more to
    taste

*1 teaspoon pepper plus more to
taste*

*2 onions and 2 celery stalks cut
in half for turkey cavities*

*1 tablespoon butter, softened to
room temperature*

*1 or 2 cups chicken broth for
basting*

¼ cup whole-wheat pastry flour

1 teaspoon Worcestershire sauce

1. Remove the oven racks except for the bottom one so that you can put the turkey on the bottom rack. Preheat the oven to 375°F.

2. Remove any giblet packages and the neck bone from the turkey cavities.

3. Rinse the turkey in cold water, including the cavities and all the skin. Pat it dry with paper towels. Put it in a large roasting pan and lightly sprinkle inside the cavities with salt and pepper. If you have a roasting pan with a rack, use the rack so that the juices and fat drip down into the pan and the turkey isn't sitting in them.

4. Turn the turkey over so that the breast is down. Put 1 onion and 1 celery stalk into the smaller cavity. Pull the skin over the cavity and secure it with metal or wooden skewers. Turn the turkey over and fold the wings underneath it. Put 1 onion and 1 celery stalk into the larger cavity.

5. Tie the drumsticks together with kitchen twine, or use the metal clamp that came with the turkey to keep the legs together. Rub the butter all over the skin with your hands. If you have a meat thermometer that isn't the instant-read kind, put it into the thickest part of the thigh, but be sure it isn't touching a bone.

6. Roast the turkey for 3 to 4 hours, depending on its size (a turkey breast may take just 1 or 2 hours). Baste with chicken broth until the turkey releases fat into the roasting pan. Then baste with the fat, every 15 to 30 minutes.

7. Start checking the meat thermometer after 2 hours. The turkey is done when the thermometer says 180°F and the juice runs clear when you poke the thigh. (Don't poke the breast, to keep all the juices in the white meat.) If the turkey is turning brown too quickly, cover it with foil while it is roasting. Keep an eye on it.

8. When the turkey is done, remove it carefully to a platter and cover it with a tent of foil. Let it sit for about 30 minutes before carving. This is when you can put all your other dishes into the oven for last-minute reheating.

9. If you want to make gravy, put the roasting pan on the stove over two burners and turn them on medium. Skim off any obvious fat with a spoon. Add broth (or water) to the roasting pan. Whisk the broth and pan drippings together with a wire whisk. Slowly add the flour and continue to whisk until the gravy reduces and thickens slightly. Season with salt, pepper, and Worcestershire sauce. Serve in a gravy boat or in a bowl with a small ladle.

~~~~~~~~ USE-WHAT-YOU-HAVE VARIATIONS ~~~~~~~~

Use any of these variations, or mix and match them according to your tastes.

VARIATION 1:   Instead of butter, try any cooking oil.

VARIATION 2:   Instead of white wine, try:
    ~ Dry (white) vermouth ~ Madeira ~ Sherry ~ Apple juice ~ White
    grape juice ~ Any broth or stock ~ Water.

VARIATION 3:   Instead of onions, celery, and carrots, in the turkey cavity, try any
    combination of:
    ~ Onions ~ Carrots ~ Leeks ~ Celery ~ Fennel ~ Parsnips.

VARIATION 4:   Instead of fresh sage and thyme, try any other fresh herbs you
    have, such as parsley, rosemary, or cilantro.

~~~~~~

Skinnygirl Rice Stuffing

This stuffing is a little different from your standard bread stuffing (although if you like that, use the recipe in *Naturally Thin* for Out of This World Stuffing). This one uses rice, so it's elegant and also nutritious. Bake this stuffing separately. *Never stuff the turkey!* It's too easy to get bacterial contamination if the stuffing doesn't get hot enough, and all the fat from the turkey soaks into the rice. Baking makes a less greasy, delicious stuffing.

Serves 12

1 tablespoon olive oil

1 large yellow onion, chopped

3 stalks celery, chopped

2 cups sliced mushrooms

Salt and pepper to taste

2 cloves garlic, minced

4 sage leaves, chopped

Leaves from 6 sprigs fresh
  thyme

¼ cup slivered almonds

¼ cup dried cranberries

½ cup white wine

1 cup vegetable broth

6 cups cooked wild rice

1 egg, lightly beaten (optional)

Parsley, for garnish

1. Preheat the oven to 350°F.

2. In a large nonstick skillet over medium heat, add the olive oil. Sauté the onion and celery until soft, 5 to 8 minutes. Add the mushrooms and continue to sauté until the mushrooms turn soft, about 5 more minutes. Add the salt and pepper. Add the garlic and cook for 1 more minute.

3. Turn off the heat and add the sage, thyme, almonds, cranberries, white wine, and vegetable broth. Stir to combine everything. Stir in the wild rice, then stir in the egg. Continue to stir until everything is completely incorporated.

4. Spray a casserole with cooking spray and put the stuffing in the casserole. Cover with a lid or foil (spray the foil with cooking spray) and bake for 30 minutes. Uncover for the last 5 or 10 minutes to brown the top slightly.

~~~~~~~~ USE-WHAT-YOU-HAVE VARIATIONS ~~~~~~~~

Use any of these variations, or mix and match them according to your tastes.

VARIATION 1:   Instead of olive oil, try any other cooking oil or butter (regular or nondairy).

VARIATION 2:   Instead of onion, try:
~ Any other kind of onion ~ 4 sliced leeks (mostly white parts) ~ 8 sliced shallots ~ 16 sliced scallions ~ ½ cup chopped chives.

VARIATION 3:   Instead of celery, try:
~ Fennel ~ Carrots ~ Parsnips ~ 1 teaspoon celery seed.

VARIATION 4:   Instead of fresh mushrooms, try baby bella mushrooms or any combination of fresh wild mushrooms.

VARIATION 5:   Instead of fresh garlic, try 1 teaspoon garlic powder or 1 teaspoon garlic salt (you won't need as much regular salt).

VARIATION 6:   Instead of fresh sage and thyme, try:
~ 1 teaspoon dried sage and 1 teaspoon dried thyme ~ Other fresh or dried herbs you have, such as parsley, rosemary, or cilantro.

VARIATION 7:   Instead of almonds and cranberries, try any combination of dried fruit (like raisins, currants, chopped apricots, cherries, chopped prunes, etc.) and nuts (walnuts, pecans, hazelnuts, etc.)

VARIATION 8:   Instead of white wine, try any broth, stock, or water.

VARIATION 9:   Instead of vegetable broth, try any other broth, stock, or water.

VARIATION 10:   Instead of wild rice, try:
~ Any other kind of rice (brown, black, red, white, jasmine, basmati, etc.) ~ Any other grain (quinoa, barley, bulgur wheat, etc.).

~~~~~~

Sweet Potato Soufflé

This recipe uses Mashed Sweet Potatoes (page 132), so make those ahead of time. Then all you have to do is whip these soufflés together and bake them while the turkey is cooling. If you don't mind beating egg whites, this recipe is ridiculously easy. Even easier, just serve the Mashed Sweet Potatoes, which are already more than amazing.

Serves 12

*4 cups mashed sweet potatoes (see the quick and easy recipe on page 132—
double it for this recipe)*
*8 egg whites, beaten until peaks are just starting to form (see Chapter 6
for how to do this)*

1. Preheat the oven to 350°F. In a bowl, mix the sweet potatoes with one-third of the beaten egg whites. Stir until completely combined. Then fold in another third. Mix until combined. Fold in the remaining egg whites and mix until combined. Stir lightly to keep air in the mixture.

2. Spray 12 ramekins or ovenproof custard cups with cooking spray. Evenly scoop the mixture into the ramekins. Place them directly on the oven rack. Bake for 30 minutes, or until the soufflés are just slightly firm to the touch. Remove them carefully so that you don't deflate them. Serve hot.

~~~~~~~~ USE-WHAT-YOU-HAVE VARIATIONS ~~~~~~~~

Use any of these variations, or mix and match them according to your tastes.

VARIATION 1:   If you don't have mashed sweet potatoes, try:
~ Butternut squash puree ~ Pumpkin puree plus ½ teaspoon cinnamon ~
Acorn squash puree ~ Regular mashed potatoes.

VARIATION 2:   Make this in a casserole dish instead of individual ramekins.

~~~~~~

Wild Rice

This traditional side dish is more nutrient dense than regular rice and it just seems to me that it should go with a holiday meal, although you could make it anytime, of course. It's very easy. You can make this recipe ahead of time, cover, refrigerate, and then just put it in the oven to reheat after you take out the turkey.

When my friend Lori tested this recipe, she used brown jasmine rice instead of wild rice and she added a slice of avocado. She said it had a Latin flair and tasted just like the rice at a hip New York restaurant called Asia de Cuba. She suggested we call it Unfried Rice. You could also make this more of a holiday rice by adding some dried cranberries and almonds, with the herbs from the Simon & Garfunkel song: parsley, sage, rosemary, and thyme.

Lori also said that the hardest part of this recipe was figuring out how long to toast the pine nuts. She burned them twice. Watch them carefully and stir them constantly in a dry skillet over medium heat until they turn golden, then remove them right away. Never leave nuts or seeds toasting on the stove or in the toaster oven when you aren't watching or they will burn.

Serves 12

2 cups wild rice, cooked according to package directions, warm
1 cup chopped fresh mint
1 cup chopped fresh basil
1 cup chopped fresh parsley
Juice from 1 lemon

4 tablespoons extra-virgin olive oil
2 teaspoons garlic salt
2 teaspoons black pepper
6 tablespoons toasted pine nuts (toast gently in a dry skillet until golden)

Put the warm rice in a serving bowl. Stir in the mint, basil, parsley, lemon juice, olive oil, garlic salt, and pepper. Taste and add more garlic salt, pepper, or lemon juice if you think they are needed. Sprinkle with the pine nuts and serve.

Use any of these variations, or mix and match them according to your tastes.

VARIATION 1:   Instead of wild rice, try any other rice or the following:
~ Orzo*~ Quinoa* ~ Couscous* ~ Spelt* ~ Bulgur wheat* ~ Barley* ~ Millet.*

(Note that other grains may require shorter cooking times.)

VARIATION 2:   Instead of mint, basil, and parsley, try any other fresh herbs, such as sage, rosemary, oregano, and thyme.

VARIATION 3:   Instead of fresh lemon juice, try any other citrus juice.

VARIATION 4:   Instead of extra-virgin olive oil, try any other good-quality cold-pressed or flavored oil.

VARIATION 5:   Instead of garlic salt, try any regular or seasoned salt.

VARIATION 6:   Instead of pine nuts, try any other chopped nuts.

~ ~

Molly Loves Corn Pudding

My former assistant Molly loves anything with corn, so I created this recipe for her. It's another traditional holiday comfort food. This version of corn pudding is not filled with cream and butter, yet it is delicious and easy. You can make and bake this dish ahead of time, then put it in the oven to warm it up along with the Wild Rice (previous recipe) after you take out the turkey.

Serves 12

½ cup raw sugar

2 cups fresh corn kernels

2 eggs plus 2 egg whites

1 cup soy milk

1½ teaspoons salt

1½ teaspoons black pepper

1 teaspoon butter (regular or nondairy)

¼ teaspoon ground nutmeg

Dash of chili powder

1. Preheat the oven to 375°F. Combine all of the ingredients in a large bowl and puree with an immersion blender, or put them all into a regular blender and puree. Leave the mixture a little chunky so that there is still some texture from the corn kernels.

2. Spray a 9 × 13-inch baking pan or casserole dish with cooking spray. Pour in the corn mixture. Bake for 1 hour, or until the mixture looks set (not liquid). Let sit for 10 minutes. Serve warm.

~~~~~~~~ USE-WHAT-YOU-HAVE VARIATIONS ~~~~~~~~

Use any of these variations, or mix and match them according to your tastes.

VARIATION 1: Instead of raw sugar, try any other dry granulated natural sweetener.

VARIATION 2: Instead of fresh corn, try frozen defrosted corn or a good brand of canned corn, drained.

VARIATION 3:   Instead of eggs and egg whites, try ²/₃ cup silken tofu.

VARIATION 4:   Instead of soy milk, try any other plain milk.

VARIATION 5:   Leave out the nutmeg.

VARIATION 6:   You could also add 1 jalapeño pepper, seeded and
minced.

~ ~

Green Bean Casserole

This delicious recipe took a few tries to get right (see Chapter 5). If you make this casserole ahead of time, don't put the fried onions on top until the final 5 minutes of reheating so that they are crispy. Finely crushing the fried onions lets you use less for the same effect.

Serves 12

1 tablespoon olive oil
½ cup diced red onion
1½ cups sliced white mushrooms
3 cups vegetable broth
5 cups haricots verts (skinny
    green beans), sliced on the
    diagonal
1 can (about 10¾ ounces) low-
    fat cream of mushroom
    soup or organic brand of
    mushroom soup (not puree—
    look for one with some
    pieces—I used Amy's brand)

½ cup soy milk
2 tablespoons reduced-fat cream
    cheese
1½ teaspoons salt
1½ teaspoons black pepper
⅓ cup canned fried onions,
    crushed

1. Put the olive oil in a large nonstick skillet with a lid or in a soup pot or Dutch oven over medium-high heat. Add the red onion and mushrooms and sauté until they turn golden, about 8 minutes. Add the vegetable broth and haricots verts. Bring the mixture to a boil, reduce the heat to medium-low, then cover and simmer for 15 minutes.

2. Uncover the pot and continue to let the beans simmer until they are soft and the broth has boiled down to about half its original volume. It doesn't have to be exact, but you really need to reduce the liquid and get the beans very tender to intensify the flavor. This could take up to 20 minutes or more.

3. Stir in the mushroom soup, soy milk, cream cheese, salt, and pepper. Mix until all of the ingredients are combined. Continue to cook for an additional 10 minutes to heat everything through and incorporate the flavors.

4. Pour the mixture into a 9 × 13-inch baking dish or casserole and bake, uncovered, for 15 minutes. Sprinkle the fried onions on top and bake for another 5 minutes. Serve hot. To warm up this casserole if you made it ahead, put it in the oven and bake until it starts to bubble. Add the onions and bake for 5 more minutes.

~~~~~~~~ USE-WHAT-YOU-HAVE VARIATIONS ~~~~~~~~

Use any of these variations, or mix and match them according to your tastes.

VARIATION 1: Instead of olive oil, try any cooking oil or butter (regular or nondairy).

VARIATION 2: Instead of red onion, try:
~ Any other kind of onion ~ Shallots, thinly sliced ~ Leeks (white parts only) ~ Scallions (mostly white parts).

VARIATION 3: Instead of white mushrooms, try any other mushrooms or mushroom mix.

VARIATION 4: Instead of vegetable broth, try any other broth, stock, or water.

VARIATION 5: Instead of fresh haricots verts, try:
~ Frozen haricots verts or French green beans ~ Regular green beans, fresh or frozen ~ Asparagus.

VARIATION 6: Instead of cream of mushroom soup, try any other low-fat white cream soup like cream of chicken or cream of broccoli.

VARIATION 7: Instead of soy milk, try any other plain milk.

VARIATION 8: Instead of reduced-fat cream cheese, try:
~ Nondairy cream cheese ~ Regular, reduced-fat, or nondairy sour cream.

VARIATION 9: Instead of fried onions, try bread crumbs or minced onions sautéed in 1 teaspoon olive oil.

~~~~~~

Chapter 14

How to Throw a Skinnygirl Party

*E*ntertaining can be stressful. You have this great idea that you are going to have a party, then you realize you have to clean, coordinate, and *cook everything*. What were you thinking? I've organized many parties, and I can tell you that throwing a party does not have to be so daunting. You can make a big impression on your guests without killing yourself if you remember these four words: *Don't be a hero*.

When I throw party, I don't stress about it because I buy the difficult items and make the easy ones. I have produced many large-scale events, and I know the secret to throwing a Skinnygirl party without letting it take over your whole week: Don't make everything from scratch. The devil is in the details. There are so many things you can buy ahead of time that you can make into something special.

Finding the Good Stuff

If you know where to look, you can find good-quality hors d'oeuvres, themed appetizers, and inexpensive but clever ways to serve them. Trader Joe's has a great selection of premade hors d'oeuvres as so do many supermarkets. Your favorite restaurants may also prepare foods for your party. Consider good Chinese, sushi, Greek, Mexican, and Italian restaurants for party ideas and themes. Purchase decor and serving accessories at local restaurants (Chinese takeout containers, chopsticks) or at stores such as IKEA, Pier 1, or Target. Some supermarkets also stock inexpensive serving ware.

Here are some ideas for purchased party food made special with a few personal touches:

- Buy frozen premade pigs in a blanket at the supermarket, with three fancy jarred mustards to dip them in. Try cranberry, wasabi, garlic, herb, horseradish, hot pepper, Dijon, whole grain, and honey flavors. Serve in ramekins.
- Order brown rice sushi rolls from a Japanese restaurant and sprinkle each roll with black sesame seeds. Serve them on inexpensive black lacquer plates.
- For a Greek theme, buy spanakopita, hummus, baba ghanoush, and baklava at a Greek restaurant or good supermarket then design your own platter of fresh and marinated vegetables. Sprinkle fresh herbs over everything.
- Men love meat. Whenever I put out platters of dried meat like prosciutto, brasaola, and pepperoni with chunks of Parmesan and crusty bread, it draws the men like a magnet. No cooking required—set out the meat and they will come.
- Buy Chinese dumplings, mini–egg rolls, and Chinese noodles from the supermarket or your favorite Chinese restaurant. Serve them in Chinese food takeout containers with chopsticks and add a big bowl of fortune cookies. Hang paper lanterns over the table.

- Buy good flavored bread, then make flavored butters to match. Mix tapenade into softened butter and you've got olive butter or add pesto, hot sauce, or honey. (See Chapter 13 for more on flavored butters.)

- Grilled pizza always impresses people. Just go to your favorite pizza place and ask for the pizza dough only. Heat up the grill, brown the underside of the pizza dough, then flip it over and top it with whatever you like. All-white cheese, grilled vegetables, and truffle oil is one of my favorite combinations. Or try leftover broccoli rabe, Parmesan, and pine nuts, and suddenly you're a big hero. This is so easy to do. Serve the pizza on a wooden cutting board with a pizza slicer so that people can help themselves. At a barbecue, you could make small pizzas on the grill and hand them out to people while you are also grilling the main course. Sprinkle with fresh herbs just before serving. You could also set up a station like an omelet bar. People put the topping they want on a plate and you make the pizzas to order.

- As I suggested in Chapter 13, buy five kinds of cheese. Make individual cheese labels and put each one on a wooden cutting board. Serve with assorted crackers and bread.

Sweet Party

Don't forget to serve something sweet, which always makes people happy. Here are some ideas:

- Hollow out fresh lemon halves, cut off the bottoms so that they are flat, arrange on a tray, and serve scoops of lemon sorbet in them. Or make them ahead and store them in egg cartons in the freezer.

- As I suggested in Chapter 13, soften low-fat vanilla ice cream and sandwich the ice cream between two cookies (purchased or home baked using any cookie recipe in this book). Wrap the sandwiches in plastic and freeze. A bunch of these look great on a platter at a party. For a pricier but quicker version, use the Carvel mini–ice-cream cookie sandwiches or ice-cream cupcakes.

- Cupcakes are more fun to eat than cake and are great for parties. Make them or buy them. Cupcake towers are easy to assemble and look impressive. You can buy inexpensive cardboard towers. I have a wrought iron cupcake tower from Bed, Bath and Beyond that I use a lot. I've also seen them on eBay. A cupcake tower provides a big "wow" factor.

Signature Cocktails

Throwing a party isn't all about the food. A lot of the charm of a great party is in the decor, music, lighting, and of course, cocktails. People love theme parties, especially when the cocktail matches the theme. My first rule for a memorable party is to create a signature cocktail (or two). Try any of the Skinnygirl cocktails in this book, or invent your own using the Skinnygirl Fixologist Formula (see Chapter 11) to get your guests into a party mood.

Typically, your guests will be happy to participate in whatever you've set as your themed cocktail. Remember to have a fun nonalcoholic option for teetotalers, and always make a pitcher or two ahead of time so that you don't spend your whole party playing bartender. Some people think those cocktail charms you hang on your glasses are cheesy, but I think they are cute and really do help people keep track of their drinks. I also like those humorous, off-color cocktail napkins. Why not give your guests something to talk (and laugh) about?

Some great signature cocktails for theme parties could be:

For Winter:

- Serve mulled wine or apple cider for a winter holiday party. Gently heat the wine or cider on low heat in a pot on the stove with whole spices like cinnamon sticks, orange peel, and whole cloves. Strain and serve in mugs.
- Serve Kir Royales for New Year's Eve: top glasses of champagne with splashes of crème de cassis.

- Serve Skinnygirl Cosmos for Valentine's Day. See the recipe on page 177, or buy the new bottled version—check www.skinnygirlcocktails.com for details.

For Spring:

- Serve Hurricanes for a Mardi Gras party. For a Skinnygirl version, put 2 ounces of rum over ice and add a splash of pineapple juice, a splash of orange liqueur (like Triple Sec), and a dash of grenadine. Fill the rest of the glass with club soda. Make them ahead of time in a pitcher (no ice) and chill.
- Forget the green beer and serve Skinnygirl Mojitos for St. Patrick's Day. See the recipe on page 173, or serve my new easy bottled version.

For Summer:

- On a hot summer day, serve Skinnygirl Piña Coladas (see the recipe in *Naturally Thin*).
- Another great summer drink: Skinnygirl Strawberry Daiquiris. Just make Skinnygirl Margaritas, but muddle a few ripe strawberries in the bottom of the glass first, then substitute clear rum for the tequila. Or, add a splash of strawberry puree if you don't have ripe strawberries.
- For a summer garden party or luncheon, serve Skinnygirl Sangria (find the recipe in *Naturally Thin*).

For Fall:

- Bloody Marys make excellent drinks for Halloween parties. You are requiring everyone come in costume, right? Make them in a punch bowl and float ice with olives frozen in it.
- Warm spiced cider, with or without the rum (see the section for winter cocktails), also makes a nice drink for a party on a chilly fall evening.

Light and Sound

Lighting and sound are some of the most important party elements. Eliminate all overhead lighting if you can. Use lamps and candles for a sexier vibe. If the lights are too bright or harsh, nobody looks good, and you don't want the conversation to turn to wrinkles and skin tone. Isn't it more fun to talk about men (or shall I say boys)? Softer lighting makes everybody feel better about themselves, which always helps the mood of a party.

The right music can totally elevate the mood in the room, but the wrong music or music turned so loud you can't hear what people are saying can wreck the party. Get the volume right. Music should be loud enough that people can hear it and sing along, but soft enough that people can still talk and hear one another. I strongly advise against launching the evening by shoving disco from the '70s down everybody's throat, even if that was "your music" back in the day. Just because it makes you nostalgic doesn't mean it makes for a classy party. Instead, start mellow, graduate to dance music, then wind down to cool jazz or lounge music.

The Food

When people are drinking, they should also be eating, if you want the party to stay under at least some reasonable control. Great food can elevate the mood and makes everybody happy. The recipes in this chapter range from finger foods to lots of fun dips, so get creative and use them as inspiration.

Grillin' and Chillin' with Phil Simms

I made this first group of Asian-inspired recipes for Phil Simms, former quarterback for the New York Giants and Super Bowl star, and his family. I'm embarrassed to say that when I was asked to cook for him, I didn't know who he was! My fiancé soon set me straight. These recipes would make a great Super Bowl party spread, or whip them up for any sports-related event. They're an elegant, healthier take on "guy food."

Beef Satay Skewers

For this recipe, you'll need 40 wooden skewers. Make them ahead of time so that the meat has time to marinate for at least 4 hours or overnight.

Makes 40 skewers

5 pounds flank steak or sirloin cut into 40 strips (the butcher can do this for you, or freeze the meat for 30 minutes so that it's easier to slice)
12 cloves garlic, chopped
8 teaspoons ground coriander
8 teaspoons honey
2 tablespoons black pepper
8 teaspoons salt
1 cup low-sodium soy sauce
8 teaspoons grated fresh ginger
4 tablespoons fresh lime juice
12 tablespoons any cooking oil
½ cup fresh chopped cilantro for garnish

1. Put the beef strips into a large plastic resealable bag or in a wide casserole dish. Mix all of the marinade ingredients (not the cilantro) together in a bowl and pour them over the meat. Cover and marinate for at least 4 hours or overnight in the refrigerator.

2. Soak 40 wooden skewers in water for at least 1 hour. Thread the beef onto the skewers. Grill or broil until done, about 5 minutes on each side. Sprinkle with the cilantro and serve with your favorite Asian or peanut sauce for dipping.

~~~~~~~~ USE-WHAT-YOU-HAVE VARIATIONS ~~~~~~~~

Use any of these variations, or mix and match them according to your tastes.

VARIATION 1: Instead of beef strips, try:
~ Chicken breast strips ~ Extra-firm tofu strips, drained and patted dry ~ Tempeh strips.

VARIATION 2: Instead of fresh garlic, try 2 tablespoons garlic powder.

VARIATION 3: Instead of ground coriander, try chopped fresh cilantro or ground cumin.

VARIATION 4: Instead of honey, try any other liquid or granulated natural sweetener.

VARIATION 5: Instead of soy sauce, try:
~ Worcestershire sauce ~ Teriyaki sauce ~ Steak sauce ~ Any storebought marinade you like.

VARIATION 6: Instead of fresh ginger, try 1 tablespoon ground ginger.

VARIATION 7: Instead of fresh lime juice, try:
~ Any other citrus juice ~ Pineapple juice ~ Any tropical juice (such as mango, passion fruit, etc.).

VARIATION 8: Instead of cilantro, try chopped fresh parsley.

~~~~~~

Simms Wasabi Tuna Sliders

These sliders make great party food because they are masculine and fun, but they'll help eliminate beer bellies. By the way, Pepperidge Farm makes whole-wheat slider buns, which I recommend for this recipe.

Serves 10 to 15

1½ cups minced scallions

3 teaspoons minced garlic

2¼ cups chopped fresh cilantro

6 tablespoons low-sodium soy sauce

3 pounds tuna steak, cut into chunks

6 tablespoons wasabi paste

3 teaspoons grated fresh ginger

6 teaspoons Dijon mustard

Salt and pepper to taste

2 teaspoons olive oil

10 to 15 small buns or rolls, preferably whole wheat

1. Combine the scallions, garlic, cilantro, and soy sauce in a bowl and mix until incorporated. Mix in the tuna until combined. Add the wasabi paste, ginger, mustard, salt, and pepper.

2. Using an ice-cream scoop, make burgers out of the mixture. Place them on a plate and chill in the refrigerator for 30 minutes.

3. Heat the olive oil in a nonstick skillet over medium-high heat. Add the tuna sliders and sauté for 5 minutes on each side. Serve on rolls with Pickled Ginger Relish (recipe follows).

~~~~~~~~~ USE-WHAT-YOU-HAVE VARIATIONS ~~~~~~~~~

Use any of these variations, or mix and match them according to your tastes.

VARIATION 1: Instead of scallions, try:

~ Any other minced onions ~ Minced shallots ~ Minced leeks, white parts only ~ Minced chives.

VARIATION 2:   Instead of garlic, try ½ teaspoon garlic powder.

VARIATION 3:   Instead of cilantro, try any other fresh leafy herb, like parsley or basil.

VARIATION 4:   Instead of soy sauce, try:
Worcestershire sauce ~ Teriyaki sauce ~ Steak sauce.

VARIATION 5:   Instead of tuna steak, try any lean ground meat or poultry.

VARIATION 6:   Instead of wasabi paste, try horseradish.

VARIATION 7:   Instead of grated fresh ginger, try ½ teaspoon ground ginger.

VARIATION 8:   Instead of Dijon mustard, try any other kind of mustard or mustard powder.

VARIATION 9:   Instead of olive oil, try any other cooking oil.

~ ~

Pickled Cucumber Ginger Relish

3 cucumbers (any kind),
   peeled, cut in half
   lengthwise and very thinly
   sliced
3 small red onions, very thinly
   sliced

6 tablespoons finely chopped
   pickled ginger
¾ cup rice vinegar
Salt and pepper to taste

In a medium bowl, thoroughly combine all of the ingredients.

Use any of these variations, or mix and match them according to your tastes.

VARIATION 1:   Instead of red onions, try any other onion, scallions, or chives.

VARIATION 2:   Instead of pickled ginger, try grated fresh gingerroot.

VARIATION 3:   Instead of rice vinegar, try any other light-colored vinegar.

~ ~

Asian Slaw

Let this tasty salad marinate for at least 3 hours or overnight. It is the perfect accompaniment to the tuna sliders and beef skewers. (The Asian Shrimp Salad on page 123 would be a nice alternative.)

Serves 10 to 15

4 teaspoons grated fresh ginger

8 teaspoons sesame oil

8 tablespoons rice vinegar

8 teaspoons soy sauce

4 teaspoons Dijon mustard

4 teaspoons minced garlic

12 tablespoons extra-virgin olive oil

1 head Napa cabbage, shredded

1 bag (about 8 ounces) shredded carrots

In a large salad bowl, whisk together the ginger, sesame oil, rice vinegar, soy sauce, mustard, garlic, and olive oil. Add the cabbage and carrots. Toss to coat, then marinate covered in the refrigerator for at least 3 hours or overnight.

Use any of these variations, or mix and match them according to your tastes.

VARIATION 1:   Instead of fresh ginger, try ½ teaspoon ground ginger.

VARIATION 2:   Instead of rice vinegar, try any other light-colored vinegar.

VARIATION 3:   Instead of Dijon mustard, try mustard powder.

VARIATION 4:   Instead of fresh garlic, try ½ teaspoon garlic powder.

VARIATION 5:   Instead of extra-virgin olive oil, try any other good-quality cold-pressed oil.

VARIATION 6:   Instead of Napa cabbage and carrots, try any combination of shredded cabbage, carrots, or coleslaw mix.

~~~~~~

Easy Dips and Spreads

A table full of dips and spreads with crackers, chips, bread, and raw vegetables can be all a cocktail party needs in the way of food. Choose from these easy dip recipes. I created the first three to make healthful, low-fat dip options for Pepperidge Farm Baked Naturals, to go with their line of crackers. Have fun with these recipes, and let them inspire you to make your own based on what you already have in your kitchen.

Simply Irresistible Blue Cheese Dip

This dip tastes so creamy and decadent, yet it's much lower in fat than the conventional version. If you love blue cheese, you are going to want to make this recipe often.

Makes about 2½ cups

8 ounces reduced-fat vegetable cream cheese, softened

1 cup reduced-fat sour cream

1 cup crumbled blue cheese

1 teaspoon garlic powder

¼ teaspoon freshly ground black pepper

1 teaspoon minced fresh parsley plus more for garnish

1 teaspoon minced fresh dill

Pepperidge Farm Baked Naturals Simply Pretzel Thins

1. Place the cream cheese, sour cream, blue cheese, garlic powder, pepper, parsley, and dill in a medium bowl. Beat with an electric mixer on medium speed until blended.

2. Sprinkle with additional parsley. Serve with pretzel thins for dipping.

~~~~~~~~ USE-WHAT-YOU-HAVE VARIATIONS ~~~~~~~~

Use any of these variations, or mix and match them according to your tastes.

VARIATION 1:   Instead of vegetable cream cheese, try any other reduced-fat plain, flavored, or nondairy cream cheese.

VARIATION 2:   Instead of sour cream, try:
~ Nondairy sour cream ~ Greek yogurt ~ Plain soy yogurt ~
Part-skim ricotta ~ Part-skim cottage cheese, whipped ~ Silken tofu plus ¼ teaspoon salt.

VARIATION 3:   Instead of blue cheese, try any other crumbly flavorful soft cheese, like feta, goat cheese, or queso fresco.

VARIATION 4:   Instead of garlic powder, try 2 cloves garlic, minced, or onion powder.

VARIATION 5:   Instead of fresh parsley and dill, try any other fresh leafy herb or herb combination.

~ ~

Lemon Basil Hummus

Tangy and tasty, this dip takes less time to make than going to the store to buy prepared hummus. It doesn't contain any tahini (sesame butter), so it's lighter than regular hummus but has the same full flavor.

Makes about 2 cups

1 can (about 16 ounces) chickpeas (garbanzo beans), drained and rinsed
½ cup fresh basil (about 5 large leaves)
1 clove garlic
1 tablespoon fresh lemon juice
1 tablespoon extra-virgin olive oil

¼ teaspoon freshly ground black pepper
1 teaspoon soy sauce
¼ teaspoon paprika
Pepperidge Farm Baked Naturals Toasted Wheat Crisps

Combine the chickpeas, basil, garlic, lemon juice, olive oil, pepper, and soy sauce in a food processor or blender and blend until smooth. Or, put these ingredients in a bowl and puree with an immersion blender. Sprinkle with the paprika and serve with the Toasted Wheat Crisps, or make ahead of time and store covered in the refrigerator.

~~~~~~~~ USE-WHAT-YOU-HAVE VARIATIONS ~~~~~~~~

Use any of these variations, or mix and match them according to your tastes.

VARIATION 1:   Instead of chickpeas, try any other white beans such as navy, cannellini, butter, great northern, etc.

VARIATION 2:   Instead of fresh basil, try any other fresh leafy herb, such as parsley or cilantro.

VARIATION 3:   Instead of garlic, try ½ teaspoon garlic powder.

VARIATION 4:   Instead of fresh lemon juice, try any other citrus juice.

VARIATION 5:   Instead of extra-virgin olive oil, try any other good-quality cold-pressed oil.

VARIATION 6:   Instead of soy sauce, try Worcestershire sauce or Teriyaki sauce.

VARIATION 7:   Instead of or in addition to garnishing with paprika, try 1 tablespoon chopped fresh parsley.

~ ~

Spicy Chipotle Dip

The third in my trio of Pepperidge Farm Baked Naturals recipes, this spicy dip is quick to make and your party guests will devour it. It has a spreadable consistency.

Makes about 2 cups

16 ounces reduced-fat chive and onion flavored cream cheese

¼ cup chipotle peppers, pureed

Juice from ½ fresh lime

Pepperidge Farm Baked Naturals Four Cheese Crisps

In a bowl mix the cream cheese, peppers, and lime together by hand, or puree with an immersion blender. Serve with the Four Cheese Crisps.

~~~~~~~~ USE-WHAT-YOU-HAVE VARIATIONS ~~~~~~~~

Use any of these variations, or mix and match them according to your tastes.

VARIATION 1:   Instead of flavored cream cheese, try:
~ Any plain reduced-fat cream cheese ~ Any reduced-fat sour cream or yogurt (this will make the recipe more like a dip and less like a spread).

VARIATION 2:   Instead of chipotle peppers, try:
~ 1–2 tablespoons chopped pickled jalapeños ~ 1 teaspoon any hot sauce ~ ¼ teaspoon cayenne pepper ~ ½ teaspoon red pepper flakes.

VARIATION 3:   Instead of fresh lime juice, try any other citrus juice.

VARIATION 4:   Instead of cheese crisps, try:
~ Baked blue corn or regular tortilla chips ~ Pretzel sticks ~ Baked potato chips ~ Toasted whole-grain pita wedges.

~~~~~~

Guilt-Free Artichoke and Spinach Dip

When I told my friend Lori that I had developed lighter versions of macaroni and cheese and chicken pot pie, she asked me to please remake "that fattening evil spinach artichoke dip" that everybody loves. This recipe was born out of that request. (My next challenge: developing a lighter version of the Cinnabon cinnamon roll—stay tuned for that in my next book.)

This is the recipe I used in the Use-What-You-Have tutorial in Chapter 4. This version of spinach artichoke dip cuts the fat way down so that you can indulge and still feel great. Don't worry about exact amounts for this recipe. If you can only find artichokes or spinach in slightly smaller or larger amounts, that's fine. Frozen is actually better than fresh because the softer texture works better for dip, so take the easy way out. Defrost the vegetables in the refrigerator overnight, then drain them in a colander in the sink or over a bowl. You can drain them together in the same colander because they'll get mixed together, anyway, and that makes fewer things to wash. After they are drained, press on them with paper towels to get rid of any extra moisture that would dilute the dip's flavor.

Another story about this recipe: Recently, I made it when shooting a segment with Isaac Mizrahi and discovered a happy accident. He didn't have an immersion blender in his kitchen, so I had to use a food processor. The food processor completely pureed the dip and I didn't need to cook it thus creating a cold dip. If you don't mind cleaning your food processor afterward, you can save time by putting everything into the food processor, pureeing, and serving. Of course, if you like your spinach artichoke dip hot, you can heat it.

Serves 6

1 package (about 9 ounces) frozen artichokes, defrosted and drained

1 package (about 9 ounces) frozen spinach, defrosted and drained

¼ cup freshly grated Parmesan cheese, divided

¼ cup shredded Monterey Jack cheese

¼ cup part-skim ricotta cheese

8 ounces reduced-fat or soy
cream cheese
2 tablespoons nondairy or
low-fat mayonnaise
½ tablespoon lemon juice

1 clove garlic, minced
¾ teaspoon salt
½ teaspoon black pepper
2 dashes Tabasco sauce

1. Preheat the oven to 350°F. Combine all of the ingredients except 2 tablespoons of the Parmesan in a large bowl or food processor. Blend or pulse until mostly smooth, but leave some artichoke chunks for texture.

2. Pour the mixture into an ovenproof dish or casserole. Sprinkle with the remaining Parmesan. Bake for 20 minutes, or until heated through and just starting to bubble. Let the dip sit for at least 10 minutes. Serve warm with thin slices of baguette, raw vegetables, baked tortilla chips, or crackers.

~~~~~~~~ USE-WHAT-YOU-HAVE VARIATIONS ~~~~~~~~

Use any of these variations, or mix and match them according to your tastes.

VARIATION 1: Instead of frozen artichokes or spinach, try:
~ Canned artichoke hearts, drained ~ Fresh spinach ~ Leaving either artichokes or spinach out and doubling the amount of the other.

VARIATION 2: Instead of Parmesan, try any other grated or shredded cheese.

VARIATION 3: Instead of Monterey Jack, try any other crumbled or shredded cheese.

VARIATION 4: Instead of ricotta, try:
~ Part-skim cottage cheese, whipped or not ~ Silken tofu.

VARIATION 5: Instead of cream cheese, try:
~ Flavorful soft goat cheese ~ Feta ~ Blue cheese.

VARIATION 6: Instead of mayonnaise, try Greek yogurt or plain soy yogurt.

VARIATION 7:   Instead of minced garlic, try:

~ ½ teaspoon garlic powder ~ ¼ teaspoon garlic or other seasoned salt (reduce other salt in recipe by ¼ teaspoon) ~ ½ teaspoon onion powder.

VARIATION 8:   Instead of Tabasco sauce, try:

~ Any other hot sauce ~ Dash of cayenne pepper ~ Pinch of red pepper flakes.

~~~~~~

Aztec Black Bean Salsa

This fresh salsa combines tender beans, crunchy onions, chewy corn, spicy jalapeño, sweet pear tomatoes, tangy lime juice, and smoky chipotle peppers. It has so much flavor that you'll probably want to make it a lot. For a party, serve with baked tortilla chips or toasted pita wedges. This also makes a great topping for a make-your-own-taco bar.

Makes about 6 cups

1 can (about 15 ounces) black
   beans, drained and rinsed
1 cup chopped red onion
1 package (about 10 ounces)
   frozen corn, defrosted and
   drained
1 tablespoon olive oil
½ fresh jalapenão pepper,
   minced
½ teaspoon salt

½ teaspoon black pepper
1 cup finely chopped pear
   tomatoes
1 chipotle pepper, minced (the
   kind in jars, with or without
   adobo sauce)
2 tablespoons chopped fresh
   cilantro
½ tablespoon fresh lime juice

1. Preheat the oven to 425°F. In a large bowl, combine the black beans, onions, corn, olive oil, jalapeño, salt, and pepper. Spread in a baking pan covered with foil. Place on the top rack of the oven and roast for 15 minutes.

2. Return the roasted vegetables to the bowl. Add the tomatoes, chipotle pepper, and cilantro. Stir to combine. Serve at room temperature.

~~~~~~~~ USE-WHAT-YOU-HAVE VARIATIONS ~~~~~~~~

Use any of these variations, or mix and match them according to your tastes.

VARIATION 1:   Instead of black beans, try any other bean (red, white, pink, etc.).

VARIATION 2:   Instead of red onion, try:
~ Any other onion ~ Chopped shallots ~ Chopped scallions, white parts and just a little of the green.

VARIATION 3:   Instead of frozen corn, try a heaping cup of fresh corn kernels.

VARIATION 4:   Instead of olive oil, try any other cooking oil.

VARIATION 5:   Instead of fresh jalapeño pepper, try:
~ Chopped mild green chilies (like Anaheim) ~ ¼ teaspoon minced poblano pepper ~ Pickled jalapeño pepper (add after roasting).

VARIATION 6:   Instead of pear tomatoes, try any other small tomato (cherry, grape) or larger chopped tomato.

VARIATION 7:   Instead of chipotle pepper, try:
~ Fresh jalapeño pepper (add before roasting) ~ Chopped mild green chilies (add before roasting) ~ ¼ teaspoon minced poblano pepper (add before roasting) ~ Pickled jalapeño pepper (add after roasting).

VARIATION 8:   Instead of fresh cilantro, try fresh parsley.

VARIATION 9:   Instead of fresh lime juice, try any other citrus juice.

~~~~~~

Low-Fat Mock-a-Mole

Increase the fiber and decrease the fat with this take on guacamole.

Makes about 1½ cups

1 avocado, peeled, pitted, and
  mashed
1 cup cooked green peas
¼ cup chopped fresh tomato
2 tablespoons chopped fresh
  cilantro plus more for garnish
1 tablespoon chopped red onion

1 tablespoon chopped fresh parsley
2 teaspoons fresh lime juice
1 teaspoon Worcestershire sauce
1 teaspoon garlic salt
½ teaspoon black pepper
¾ teaspoon Tabasco sauce

Combine all of the ingredients in a large bowl and blend with an immersion blender until smooth. You can garnish with cilantro. Serve with tortilla chips, whole grain crackers, and raw vegetables.

~~~~~~~~ USE-WHAT-YOU-HAVE VARIATIONS ~~~~~~~~

Use any of these variations, or mix and match them according to your tastes.

VARIATION 1: Instead of cooked peas, try an additional avocado.

VARIATION 2: Instead of tomato, try chopped pear, grape, or cherry tomatoes.

VARIATION 3: Instead of cilantro, try doubling the amount of parsley.

VARIATION 4: Instead of red onion, try:
~ Any other onion ~ Scallions, white parts and some of the green ~ Chives.

VARIATION 5: Instead of fresh parsley, try adding 1 extra tablespoon fresh cilantro.

VARIATION 6: Instead of fresh lime juice, try any other citrus juice.

VARIATION 7: Instead of Worcestershire sauce, try soy sauce (including tamari or shoyu).

VARIATION 8: Instead of garlic salt, try:
~ 1 Clove garlic, minced, plus ¾ teaspoon regular or seasoned salt.

VARIATION 9: Instead of Tabasco sauce, try:
~ Any other hot sauce ~ 1 dash cayenne pepper ~ 1 pinch red pepper flakes.

~ ~

Herbed Goat Cheese Dip

This is another superquick dip that tastes like a gourmet snack.

Makes about ¾ cup

6 ounces goat cheese

2 sun-dried tomatoes, soaked in water, drained, and chopped

1 teaspoon dried tarragon

⅛ teaspoon black pepper

Stir the goat cheese, sun-dried tomatoes, tarragon, and pepper together in a small bowl. Serve with crackers for dipping.

~ ~ ~ ~ ~ ~ ~ ~ USE-WHAT-YOU-HAVE VARIATIONS ~ ~ ~ ~ ~ ~ ~ ~

Use any of these variations, or mix and match them according to your tastes.

VARIATION 1: Instead of goat cheese, try:
~ Any reduced-fat regular or nondairy cream cheese ~ Greek yogurt (for a more diplike consistency).

VARIATION 2:   Instead of sun-dried tomatoes, try:

~ 2 plum tomatoes, seeded and minced ~ Chopped black or green olives.

VARIATION 3:   Instead of dried tarragon, try:

~ 1 tablespoon chopped fresh tarragon ~ 1 tablespoon chopped fresh basil ~ ½ teaspoon dried rosemary ~ ½ teaspoon dried oregano ~ ½ teaspoon dried thyme.

VARIATION 4:   Instead of crackers, try:

~ Toasted pita wedges ~ Flatbread wedges ~ Slices of toasted baguette ~ Whole-grain baked tortilla chips.

~ ~

Homemade Salsa

You can always find a pretty good salsa in the store and doctor it, but salsa is so easy to make that I recommend trying it at home at least once. You can be creative with salsa, and it's a great way to use what you have. Try adding corn, black beans, bell peppers, or different herbs. Here is a very basic recipe to get you started. The adornments are up to you. This makes about 2 to 3 cups, depending on the size of your tomatoes.

2 large tomatoes, or 4 to 6 plums tomatoes

1 medium white onion, coarsely chopped

½ to 1 jalapeño pepper

Juice from ½ fresh lime or lemon

Salt and pepper to taste

Fresh chopped cilantro

Combine the tomatoes, onion, jalapeño, and lime juice in a blender. Pulse until mostly smooth. Pour into a bowl, add salt and pepper to taste, and sprinkle with the cilantro. To make pico de gallo, just chop everything with a knife rather than blend. How easy is that?

※

What-the-Hell-Do-I-Do-with-These-Leftover-Avocados Dip

Yes, I had leftover avocados when I created this dip and avocados are so versatile. It was a use-what-you-have moment. I knew I had to do something with those avocados sitting on my counter, so this is what I did. It's a little bit different from basic guacamole.

Makes about 3 to 4 cups

1 cup chopped tomatoes

3 avocados, halved, pitted, scored into cubes, and removed with a spoon

1 cup fresh corn kernels

1 teaspoon salt

1 teaspoon black pepper

2 chipotle peppers, chopped

1 teaspoon Tabasco sauce

½ teaspoon ground cumin

2 tablespoons chopped fresh parsley

1 teaspoon fresh lemon juice

Combine all of the ingredients in a bowl and mix and mash to your desired texture. Serve with baked tortilla chips.

~~~~~~~~ USE-WHAT-YOU-HAVE VARIATIONS ~~~~~~~~

Use any of these variations, or mix and match them according to your tastes.

VARIATION 1: Instead of fresh corn kernels, try:
~ Leftover grilled or roasted corn ~ Frozen defrosted corn, drained ~ Canned corn, rinsed and drained.

VARIATION 2:   Instead of chipotle peppers, try any other hot pepper or pepperoncini, such as jalapeño, poblano, Anaheim, etc.

VARIATION 3:   Instead of Tabasco sauce, try:
~ Any other hot sauce ~ ¼ teaspoon cayenne pepper ~ ¼ teaspoon red pepper flakes.

VARIATION 4:   Instead of cumin, try chili powder or Worcestershire sauce.

VARIATION 5:   Instead of fresh parsley, try any other fresh leafy herb, such as cilantro.

VARIATION 6:   Instead of fresh lemon juice, try any other citrus juice.

VARIATION 7:   Instead of serving this dip on chips, try:
~ Whole-grain crackers ~ Baked pita wedges ~ Any other sturdy dipping cracker or chip.

~ ~

Chapter 15

Top Chefs, Skinnygirl Recipes

Throughout my colorful career, I've been fortunate enough to meet so many interesting people. Many of those people have been great chefs. I asked some of them for their favorite recipes, which also happen to be good for you. This chapter contains those recipes from a few of my extremely talented chef friends and peers—the inimitable Bobby Flay, and three of my friends from the Bravo series *Top Chef*, Lee Anne Wong from the first season of *Top Chef*, and Ariane Duarte and Hosea Rosenberg from the fifth season.

Each has a unique style and embraces healthy cooking in a personal way. Although these recipes aren't mine, I've edited a few of them just slightly in keeping with the Skinnygirl style.

These chefs are cooking at a level that I rarely attain. They can hack up chickens and fillet fish in the time it takes me to make a Skinnygirl Margarita. They have restaurants and I don't. Their recipes are a little more complicated than the ones I've given you in this book, but if you've been through this book and read about the techniques, and if you feel confident, you are ready for them.

This chapter takes cooking up a notch, with some new gourmet foodie terms and some new techniques. Frankly, I've learned some new terms from my chef friends, too. Even so, none of these recipes are difficult, and they are all in keeping with the Skinnygirl style. You're going to gain a chef's confidence once you give them a try. You'll also blow your guests or your family away. *You*, the one who they thought couldn't cook.

So that you can continue to practice and learn how to use what you have, I've included my own Use-What-You-Have Variations for these recipes. Be forewarned that any substitutions are not what the chef originally intended—most good chefs are very particular.

Bobby Flay

Bobby Flay is one of the most well-known chefs in America today. He is a restaurateur, award-winning cookbook author, and TV star, and a friendly, generous person, too. His first restaurant was the famous Mesa Grill in New York City, and he's opened up other Mesa Grills in the Bahamas and Las Vegas. He's also got a steak house in Atlantic City, Bar Americain in New York City, and Bobby's Burger Palace, with locations in New York, New Jersey, and Connecticut. Thanks, Bobby, for sharing these delicious recipes! Find out more about Bobby Flay at www.bobbyflay.com.

Spanish Spiced Rubbed Chicken with Mustard-Green Onion Sauce

This recipe has several parts, but they aren't complicated. You can make the sauce and the spice rub ahead of time, then put it all together quickly. Bobby is all about grilling, but he also gives the option to make this on the stove, as you'll see in the recipe.

Serves 4

Olive oil

4 boneless, skinless chicken
    breasts (about 6 ounces each)

Kosher salt

Spanish Spice Rub (recipe
    follows)

Mustard–Green Onion Sauce
    (recipe follows)

Chopped fresh parsley for
    garnish

1. Heat the grill to medium-high (spray with cooking spray or oil the grill grate) or heat 2 tablespoons of olive oil in a large nonstick sauté pan.

2. Season each chicken breast with salt on both sides. Rub each breast on the top side with the rub and place on the grill or in the pan, rub side down. Cook for about 3 minutes, or until slightly charred and a crust has formed. Turn the breasts over and continue cooking for about 5 more minutes, or until just cooked through.

3. Spoon some of the Mustard–Green Onion Sauce onto a platter and place the breasts on top. Garnish with the parsley and serve the remaining sauce on the side.

~~~~~~~~~ USE-WHAT-YOU-HAVE VARIATIONS ~~~~~~~~~

Use any of these variations, or mix and match them according to your tastes.

VARIATION 1:   Instead of chicken breasts, try:
   ~ Your favorite cut of beef ~ Pork tenderloins ~ Salmon steaks ~4-ounce slices extra-firm tofu, drained (marinate in the rub).

VARIATION 2:   Instead of kosher salt, try regular salt.

VARIATION 3:   Instead of olive oil, try any other cooking oil.

VARIATION 4:   Instead of parsley, try chopped fresh cilantro.

~~~~~~

For the Spanish Spice Rub

1½ tablespoons Spanish paprika
   (pimentón)
1½ teaspoons ground cumin
1½ teaspoons ground mustard
   powder

1 teaspoon ground fennel
1 teaspoon coarsely ground
   black pepper
1 teaspoon kosher salt

Whisk together all of the ingredients in a bowl.

~~~~~~~~ USE-WHAT-YOU-HAVE VARIATIONS ~~~~~~~~

Use any of these variations, or mix and match them according to your tastes.

VARIATION 1:   Instead of Spanish paprika, try any other kind of paprika or chili powder.

VARIATION 2:   Instead of ground cumin, try:
~ Cumin seeds, ground in a spice grinder ~ Ground coriander or coriander seeds ground in a spice grinder.

VARIATION 3:   Instead of ground mustard powder, try:
~ 1 teaspoon wasabi powder ~ 1 teaspoon horseradish powder ~ Mustard seeds, ground in a spice grinder ~ 1 tablespoon prepared mustard (then you will need to spread the rub because it will be a paste, not a powder).

VARIATION 4:   Instead of ground fennel, try crushed caraway seeds or ½ teaspoon anise seeds.

VARIATION 5:   Instead of kosher salt, try regular salt.

~~~~~~

Mustard-Green Onion Sauce

¼ cup aged white wine vinegar

2 tablespoons Dijon mustard

1 teaspoon clover honey

½ cup plus 2 tablespoons extra-
   virgin olive oil

Salt and freshly ground pepper
   to taste

¼ cup thinly sliced green onions

3 tablespoons finely chopped
   fresh flat-leaf parsley

Whisk together the vinegar, mustard, and honey in a large bowl. Slowly whisk in the olive oil until emulsified and season with salt and pepper. Fold in the green onions and parsley.

~~~~~~~~ USE-WHAT-YOU-HAVE VARIATIONS ~~~~~~~~

Use any of these variations, or mix and match them according to your tastes.

VARIATION 1:   Instead of aged white wine vinegar, try any good-quality light-colored vinegar such as champagne vinegar.

VARIATION 2:   Instead of Dijon mustard, try any other kind of mustard or 2 teaspoons ground mustard powder.

VARIATION 3:   Instead of clover honey, try any other natural liquid sweetener.

VARIATION 4:   Instead of extra-virgin olive oil, try any other good-quality cold-pressed oil.

VARIATION 5:   Instead of fresh flat-leaf parsley, try fresh cilantro.

~~~~~~~~~~~~~~~~~~~~~~~~~~~~~~~~~~~~~~

Grilled Basil-Rubbed Pork Chops with Grilled Nectarine–Blue Cheese Salad and Toasted Pignoli Nuts

Can something this elegant be this easy? Oh yes. You have to try this recipe.

Serves 4

*4 center-cut boneless pork chops
(about 6 ounces each)
8 basil leaves*

*Olive oil
Salt and pepper to taste*

Preheat the grill or grill pan over high heat. Rub both sides of each pork chop with basil, brush with olive oil, and season with salt and pepper. Grill for about 4 minutes per side, or until slightly charred and just cooked through. Remove to a plate and let rest a few minutes before serving.

~~~~~~~~~ USE-WHAT-YOU-HAVE VARIATIONS ~~~~~~~~~

Use any of these variations, or mix and match them according to your tastes.

VARIATION 1:   Instead of pork chops, try:

~ Chicken breasts ~ Salmon steaks ~ 4-ounce slices extra-firm tofu, drained.

VARIATION 2:   Instead of basil, try any other fresh leafy herb.

VARIATION 3:   Instead of olive oil, try canola oil or peanut oil.

~~~~~~

For the Grilled Nectarine-Blue Cheese Salad

4 nectarines, slightly
　　underripe, halved
Olive oil
¼ pound blue cheese,
　　crumbled
2 tablespoons honey
8 basil leaves, sliced into thin
　　ribbons

2 tablespoons toasted pine
　　nuts (toast gently in
　　a dry skillet until
　　golden)
Coarsely ground black
　　pepper to taste

1. Heat the grill or grill pan over high heat. Brush the cut side of the nectarines with olive oil and place on the grill, cut side down. Grill for 2 to 3 minutes, or until golden brown and caramelized. Turn over and grill about 2 minutes longer, or until slightly soft and just warmed through.

2. Remove the nectarines from the grill and top each half with some of the blue cheese. Drizzle with honey and garnish with basil, pine nuts, and a sprinkling of pepper.

~~~~~~~~ USE-WHAT-YOU-HAVE VARIATIONS ~~~~~~~~

Use any of these variations, or mix and match them according to your tastes.

VARIATION 1:　Instead of nectarines, try:
~ Peaches ~ 8 plums ~ 8 apricots ~ Apples, cored and halved ~ Pears, cored and halved.

VARIATION 2:　Instead of olive oil, try any other cooking oil or melted butter (regular or nondairy).

VARIATION 3:　Instead of blue cheese, try any other crumbled cheese with a lot of flavor.

VARIATION 4:　Instead of honey, try any other natural liquid sweetener.

VARIATION 5: Instead of basil leaves, try:

~ ½ teaspoon crumbled dried basil ~ Fresh mint leaves ~ ¼ teaspoon ground cinnamon.

~ ~

Slow-Roasted Salmon with Herb Vinaigrette

Bobby says to use two individual-size cazuelas in this recipe, but you probably don't have these South American cooking pots. Honestly, I didn't even know what these were until I looked up the word. Maybe that's why Bobby Flay has a thousand restaurants and I don't have any. For the purposes of this recipe, a cazuela is just a baking dish (now I know!). Any casserole dish can substitute, so if you have individual-size casserole dishes or stoneware or clay crocks about 8 inches in diameter, those would be fine. If you only have one larger casserole or baking dish, you can make this in one pot instead of two.

Serves 2

Olive oil

1½ medium Idaho potatoes, peeled and sliced into ¼-inch-thick slices

Kosher salt and freshly ground black pepper to taste

2 salmon fillets (about 6 ounces each)

¼ cup red wine vinegar

1 teaspoon Dijon mustard

1 small clove garlic, finely chopped

½ teaspoon finely chopped fresh rosemary

½ teaspoon finely chopped fresh sage

½ teaspoon finely chopped fresh thyme

1 tablespoon finely chopped fresh parsley

6 tablespoons extra-virgin olive oil

1. Preheat the oven to 400°F. Brush two 8-inch cazuelas with olive oil and arrange the potato slices in one layer in the bottom. Brush the potatoes with olive oil and season with salt and pepper. Bake in the oven for 12 to 15 minutes, or until lightly golden brown and slightly soft. Remove the potatoes and reduce the oven temperature to 250°F.

2. Season the salmon with salt and pepper and place the fillets on top of the potatoes, skin side up. Roast in the oven to medium doneness, 12 to 14 minutes.

3. While the salmon is roasting, whisk together the vinegar, mustard, garlic, and herbs in a medium bowl. Slowly whisk in the olive oil until well-combined and season with salt and pepper to taste.

4. Remove the salmon and potatoes from the oven and immediately drizzle each fillet with some of the vinaigrette.

~~~~~~~~ USE-WHAT-YOU-HAVE VARIATIONS ~~~~~~~~

Use any of these variations, or mix and match them according to your tastes.

VARIATION 1:   Instead of Idaho potatoes, try any other potato.

VARIATION 2:   Instead of olive oil for the cazuelas, try any other cooking oil or melted butter (regular or nondairy).

VARIATION 3:   Instead of kosher salt, try regular salt.

VARIATION 4:   Instead of salmon fillets, try:
~ Chicken breasts* ~ Chicken legs or thighs* ~ Lamb or veal shanks* ~ Pork chops* ~ 4-ounce slices extra-firm tofu, drained.

VARIATION 5:   Instead of red wine vinegar, try any other good vinegar or citrus juice.

VARIATION 6:   Instead of Dijon mustard, try any other kind of mustard or ¼ teaspoon ground mustard powder.

* Will probably require longer cooking time depending on your desired degree of doneness.

VARIATION 7:   Instead of garlic clove, try ½ teaspoon garlic powder or ½ teaspoon minced fresh ginger.

VARIATION 8:   Instead of fresh rosemary, sage, thyme, and parsley, try any other fresh herbs.

VARIATION 9:   Instead of extra-virgin olive oil for the vinaigrette, try any nut oil or other good-quality cold-pressed oil.

~ ~

Lee Anne Wong

Lee Anne Wong was the fan favorite on season 1 of *Top Chef* and she's still very involved in the Bravo TV family. She happens to cook very healthful food. These recipes would be excellent choices for any intimate Skinnygirl dinner. Lee Anne uses some exotic Asian ingredients in her cooking, such as yuzu, ponzu, and kombu. As I write this, I swear I have no idea what sudachi is, but Lee Anne obviously knows. You should be able to find all of these in any Asian market and even in some gourmet or health food stores that sell ethnic foods.

JULIE-WHO?

The term *julienne* means to cut into thin sticks, like matchsticks. It's a common preparation for carrots, radishes, and other firm vegetables. It looks nice, so chefs use it frequently. It's easy to julienne at home and will add to your presentation. Just cut the vegetable into the length you want (usually 1 or 2 inches), slice, then cut the slices into thin strips. Honestly, though, I don't usually have the patience.

Steamed Bass with Root Vegetable Salad and Ponzu Sauce

Don't let these recipes scare you! A few of them have some unusual ingredients that you might not have heard of before. You may have a hard time finding them unless you take your shopping list to an Asian grocery store (specifically a Japanese grocery store). If you can't or you don't have access to an Asian grocery store, don't worry. The Use-What-You-Have Variations following the recipes will give you options that are easier to find. I urge you to try these, even if you are substituting a lot of ingredients. They will still be delicious.

Serves 4

4 boneless, skinless bass fillets
(about 5 ounces each)
1 tablespoon yuzu juice (an
Asian citrus juice)
2 tablespoons vegetable oil
Salt and white pepper to taste
Banana leaf for wrapping

8 shiso leaves
4 pieces scallion, julienned into
2-inch matchsticks, white
and green parts
2-inch piece of fresh ginger,
peeled and julienned into
2-inch matchsticks

1. Rinse and pat the fish fillets dry. In a small bowl, whisk together the yuzu juice and vegetable oil. Brush both sides of each fillet with the vinaigrette. Season lightly with salt and pepper.

2. Cut pieces of the banana leaf large enough to wrap each fillet completely. Place a piece of shiso on the banana leaf. Place the fish fillet on top of the shiso and top with another shiso leaf. Top the fillets with a generous pinch of scallion and ginger. Carefully wrap each fillet in the banana leaf to make a package and tie securely with butcher's twine.

3. Place the packets in a steam basket approximately 3 inches over boiling water. Cover with a tight-fitting lid. Steam the fillets for 8 minutes, until just cooked through. Unwrap the fish and discard the shiso leaves, scallion, and ginger. Serve immediately with Root Vegetable Salad and Ponzu Sauce (recipes follow).

~~~~~~~~ USE-WHAT-YOU-HAVE VARIATIONS ~~~~~~~~

Use any of these variations, or mix and match them according to your tastes.

VARIATION 1:   Instead of bass fillets, try:
~ Red snapper ~ Tilapia ~ Sea bass ~ Halibut ~ Monkfish ~ Salmon ~ Extra-firm tofu slices, drained and patted dry.

VARIATION 2:   Instead of yuzu juice, try:
~ Fresh lemon juice mixed with fresh lime juice ~ Fresh lemon juice ~ Fresh lime juice ~ Fresh grapefruit juice.

VARIATION 3:   Instead of the banana leaf, try parchment paper.

VARIATION 4:   Instead of shiso leaves, try fresh basil leaves or fresh mint leaves.

~~~~~~

Root Vegetable Salad

All the root vegetables in this recipe are raw. They are julienned into matchsticks and they are delicious. If you've never tried a raw beet or a raw sweet potato, this is your chance.

CHIFFONADE

To chiffonade means to cut into long, very thin strips—much thinner than the matchstick you would use for the julienne technique. Typically, a chiffonade is for leafy vegetables or herbs such as spinach, kale, basil, or in the case of the following recipe, shiso. Stack the leaves and roll them up as tightly as you can. Then, with a sharp knife, cut them into very thin ribbons. It's a beautiful technique that can add the *wow* factor to your presentation.

1 red beet, peeled	*1 teaspoon yuzu juice*
1 daikon or watermelon radish,	*¼ teaspoon sugar*
peeled	*1 tablespoon shiso leaf, cut into*
1 sweet potato, peeled	*a fine chiffonade*
1 tablespoon olive oil	*Salt and black pepper to taste*

1. Julienne all of the root vegetables to ⅛-inch-thick matchsticks, about 3 inches in length.

2. Combine the olive oil, yuzu juice, and sugar in a bowl, whisking until the sugar dissolves.

3. Toss the vegetables and shiso leaf in the vinaigrette and season generously with salt and pepper. Serve immediately on top of the steamed fish fillet, drizzled with Ponzu Sauce (recipe follows).

~~~~~~~~ USE-WHAT-YOU-HAVE VARIATIONS ~~~~~~~~

Use any of these variations, or mix and match them according to your tastes.

VARIATION 1: Instead of red beet, try:
~ Any other kind of beet ~ Parsnip ~ Turnip.

VARIATION 2: Instead of daikon or watermelon radish, try:
~ Regular radish ~ Jicama ~ Kohlrabi, peeled (a radishlike vegetable).

VARIATION 3: Instead of sweet potato, try:
~ Butternut squash, peeled ~ Acorn squash, peeled ~ Carrot.

VARIATION 4: Instead of yuzu juice, try:
~ Fresh lemon juice mixed with fresh lime juice ~ Fresh lemon juice ~ Fresh lime juice ~ Fresh grapefruit juice.

VARIATION 5: Instead of shiso leaves, try fresh basil leaves or fresh mint leaves.

~~~~~~

Ponzu Sauce

This tart-and-salty sauce has an amazing and unique taste, even if you have to substitute some things. Mirin is a sweet Japanese cooking wine and you sometimes get bonito flakes on sushi rolls. Kombu is a sea vegetable. All these should be available in an Asian grocery store, but if you can't find them, see the Use-What-You-Have Variations.

1 cup sudachi juice
⅓ cup plus 2 tablespoons rice
    vinegar
1 cup plus 2 tablespoons soy
    sauce

3 tablespoons mirin
1 tablespoon dried bonito flakes
1 piece kombu, cut into a 2-inch
    square

Mix all of the ingredients together in a bowl and refrigerate for 24 hours. Strain the solids through a fine cheesecloth. Drizzle the sauce over the fish.

~~~~~~~~ USE-WHAT-YOU-HAVE VARIATIONS ~~~~~~~~

Use any of these variations, or mix and match them according to your tastes.

VARIATION 1:   Instead of sudachi juice, try:
~ Fresh lemon juice mixed with fresh lime juice ~ Fresh lemon juice ~ Fresh lime juice ~ Fresh grapefruit juice.

VARIATION 2:   Instead of rice vinegar, try champagne vinegar or ⅓ cup white vinegar plus 2 tablespoons apple juice or water.

VARIATION 3:   Instead of mirin, try:
~ 2 tablespoons white wine plus 1 tablespoon sugar, honey, or agave nectar (stir to dissolve) ~ 2 tablespoons cooking sherry plus 1 tablespoon sugar, honey, or agave nectar (stir to dissolve).

VARIATION 4: Instead of dried bonito flakes, try:

~ Fish sauce ~ Shrimp stock or broth ~ 1 teaspoon clam juice ~ Vegetable bouillon cube or granules.

VARIATION 5: Instead of kombu, try:

~ ½ teaspoon fish sauce ~ ½ teaspoon kelp powder ~ Another sea vegetable, such as dulse or wakame ~ ½ teaspoon anchovy paste.

~ ~

Seared Diver Scallops, Summer Succotash, and Orange Gastrique

This amazing scallop recipe calls for diver scallops, which are scallops that divers actually harvest by hand. They tend to be higher in quality and certainly they are environmentally friendlier. However, any good scallops will do. U-12 means that there are twelve scallops in a pound. These are relatively small scallops. This recipe seems kind of complicated, but it's really not. Just get all of your ingredients ready before you start (remember the *mise en place* rule) and it all comes together quickly. The results are stunning.

Serves 4

12 diver scallops (U-12)

Salt and white pepper to taste

1 tablespoon butter

1 cup fresh corn kernels

1 cup cooked shell beans, such as favas or limas

1 clove garlic, minced

¼ cup diced red bell pepper

¼ cup scallions, sliced crosswise

Juice of ½ lemon

3 tablespoons julienned fresh basil

1 tablespoon julienned fresh mint

1 tablespoon minced fresh parsley

12 orange segments (cut off all
   the peel and white pith)
Sugar for dusting
1 cup raw sugar
½ cup rice vinegar
½ teaspoon red pepper flakes
1 cup fresh orange juice

2 tablespoons extra-virgin olive
   oil
Pea tendrils or baby arugula for
   garnish
Fresh lemon juice
Extra-virgin olive oil

1. Rinse and pat the scallops dry and leave out at room temperature for 5 minutes. Season generously with salt and pepper.

2. To make the succotash, in a large nonstick skillet, melt the butter over high heat. Add the corn kernels and sauté for 3 minutes, or until tender. Add the cooked beans and cook for 2 more minutes. Add the garlic, red bell pepper, and scallions, and cook for 3 more minutes. Season well with salt and pepper and stir in the lemon juice, basil, mint, and parsley. Keep warm until needed.

3. Lay the orange segments on a baking sheet and lightly sprinkle with sugar. Put them under the broiler for 1 minute to caramelize the sugar. (Lee Anne uses a blowtorch to do this, but I am going to assume you don't have one of those!)

4. In a saucepan, combine 1 cup sugar, rice vinegar, red pepper flakes, and orange juice. Bring to a boil over high heat. Cook until the gastrique has reduced to about 1 cup and thickened into a syrup, about 10 minutes. Cool completely before using.

5. Heat 1 tablespoon of olive oil in a 12-inch nonstick skillet over medium-high heat until hot but not smoking, then sear 6 scallops, turning once, until golden brown on both sides and just cooked through, 2 to 4 minutes total. Trans-

GASTRIQUE

A gastrique is a vinegar–sugar mixture that is heated until it is reduced to a syrup. It is then added to sauce for flavoring meat or fish, often in conjunction with fruit. In the Seared Diver Scallops recipe, the gastrique and orange give the scallops a delicious flavor.

fer to a platter and keep warm, loosely covered with foil. Sear the remaining scallops in the same manner, wiping out the skillet and adding about 1 tablespoon of olive oil between batches.

6. To serve, divide the succotash between four plates. Place 3 scallops on each plate and top each scallop with the prepared orange segments. Lightly dress the pea tendrils or arugula with a few drops of lemon juice and extra-virgin olive oil, salt and pepper, tossing to coat. Drizzle the gastrique around the plate and garnish with the dressed greens. Serve immediately.

~~~~~~~~ USE-WHAT-YOU-HAVE VARIATIONS ~~~~~~~~

Use any of these variations, or mix and match them according to your tastes.

VARIATION 1:   Instead of scallops, try:
~ Shrimp ~ "Tofu scallops" made out of extra-firm tofu (cut it into circles so that it is in the same shape as a scallop).

VARIATION 2:   Instead of butter, try:
~ Soy butter ~ Olive oil ~ Peanut oil.

VARIATION 3:   Instead of fresh corn, try frozen defrosted corn, drained.

VARIATION 4:   Instead of garlic, try ½ teaspoon garlic powder.

VARIATION 5:   Instead of red bell pepper, try jarred roasted red pepper.

VARIATION 6:   Instead of fresh lemon juice, try fresh lime juice.

VARIATION 7:   Instead of fresh basil, mint, and parsley, try any other fresh herbs.

VARIATION 8:   Instead of orange segments, try tangerine segments or grapefruit segments.

VARIATION 9:   Instead of rice vinegar, try champagne vinegar or white wine vinegar.

VARIATION 10:   Instead of pea tendrils or baby arugula, try any fresh baby green or spring green mixture.

~~~~~~~~~~~~~~~~~~~~~~~~~~~~~~~~~~~~~~~

Seared Watermelon Salad with Roasted Tomatoes and Arugula

This recipe has an impressive presentation with the stacks of watermelon and tomato with goat cheese between them. You'll feel like you're at an upscale spa, even though the recipe is easy. When the tomatoes are roasting, you can do something else, so this recipe doesn't take constant babysitting, and the assembly part at the end is fun.

Serves 4

4 plum tomatoes

1 teaspoon salt

½ tablespoon finely chopped
   fresh rosemary

½ tablespoon finely chopped
   fresh thyme

½ tablespoon finely chopped
   fresh chervil

¼ cup olive oil

Salt and freshly ground black
   pepper

Half of a seedless watermelon

4 ounces goat cheese

2 tablespoons milk

Vegetable oil for frying

4 cups arugula

¼ cup Tomato-Watermelon
   Vinaigrette (recipe follows)

1. Preheat the oven to 225°F. Slice the plum tomatoes in half and place on a parchment-lined baking sheet, cut side facing up.

2. In a small bowl, combine 1 teaspoon salt, rosemary, thyme, and chervil. Brush the tomatoes with the olive oil and sprinkle generously with the salt and herb mixture. Season with the pepper. Place the tomatoes in the oven and cook for 1 hour. Remove from the oven and allow to cool to room temperature.

3. Cut the watermelon into ½-inch-thick slices. Using a 3-inch round cookie cutter or a biscuit cutter, cut out 12 pieces of watermelon. Set aside, refrigerated, until needed.

4. In a small bowl, whisk together the goat cheese and milk until it is a smooth consistency. This may also be achieved in a food processor. Place the goat cheese in a pastry bag with a fluted tip. Refrigerate until needed. Let the goat cheese stand at room temperature 15 minutes prior to serving time, to allow the cheese to soften slightly.

5. Heat a large nonstick sauté pan over high heat with enough vegetable oil to lightly coat the bottom of the pan. Season both sides of the watermelon slices with salt and pepper. When the pan is barely smoking, carefully add the watermelon slices (you may have to cook in several batches). Do not crowd the pan. The watermelon will react with the oil, so be careful of oil splashes. Sear the watermelon over high heat until it has caramelized, about 1 minute, then flip and cook on the other side for 1 minute more. Remove the watermelon and drain on paper towels. Repeat with the remaining melon slices.

6. To serve, toss the arugula with the Tomato–Watermelon Vinaigrette. Season to taste with salt and pepper. Beginning with a watermelon slice, pipe a small amount (¼ ounce) of goat cheese on top of the melon. Layer with a roasted tomato piece, then more goat cheese, then melon, goat cheese, tomato, goat cheese, and top with a third piece of melon. Lay the stack horizontally and serve immediately with the dressed arugula.

~~~~~~~~ USE-WHAT-YOU-HAVE VARIATIONS ~~~~~~~~

Use any of these variations, or mix and match them according to your tastes.

VARIATION 1:   Instead of fresh rosemary, thyme, and chervil, try any other fresh herbs.

VARIATION 2:   Instead of goat cheese, try any other crumbled cheese.

VARIATION 3:   Instead of piping the goat cheese with a pastry bag, just spoon it on.

VARIATION 4:   Instead of milk, try any other plain milk.

VARIATION 5:   Instead of arugula, try any other fresh leafy greens.

~~~~~~

Tomato-Watermelon Vinaigrette

1 tablespoon olive oil

1 clove garlic, finely chopped

1 teaspoon minced fresh
ginger

1 plum tomato, peeled,
seeded, and diced

½ cup watermelon, seeded and
diced into ¼-inch pieces

½ teaspoon finely chopped fresh
rosemary

1 teaspoon salt

2 teaspoons sugar

3 tablespoons champagne
vinegar

¾ cup vegetable oil

Salt and pepper to taste

1. In a medium nonstick sauté pan, heat the olive oil over medium heat. Add the garlic and ginger and cook until fragrant and lightly colored, about 1 minute.

2. Add the diced tomato, watermelon, rosemary, 1 teaspoon salt, and sugar. Continue to cook over medium heat, stirring often, for about 5 minutes, until the tomato and watermelon have softened and broken down. Allow to cool to room temperature.

3. Add the tomato–melon mixture to a food processor or blender with the champagne vinegar. (You can also use an immersion blender.) Process the mixture until smooth, adding the vegetable oil while blending in a thin, steady stream to form an emulsification. Season with salt and pepper. Refrigerate until needed.

~~~~~~~~ USE-WHAT-YOU-HAVE VARIATIONS ~~~~~~~~

Use any of these variations, or mix and match them according to your tastes.

VARIATION 1: Instead of the plum tomato, try half of a regular tomato or a sun-dried tomato, soaked in warm water to plump it, then minced.

VARIATION 2: Instead of fresh rosemary, try any other fresh herbs.

VARIATION 3: Instead of champagne vinegar, try rice vinegar.

~~~~~~

Ariane Duarte

Ariane was the sleeper hit on season 5 of *Top Chef*. Everybody loved her—and called her "the Cougar." Ariane owns her own restaurant, Culin-Ariane, in New Jersey, with her husband, Michael. Ariane is a gifted chef with a knack for bringing out amazing flavors in good ingredients. She was kind enough to share her very simple recipes for a complete dinner that will impress your guests. The Creamy Cauliflower Puree is the same recipe that won the *Today* show challenge on *Top Chef*. Find out more about Ariane and her restaurant at culinariane.com.

Orange Juice Brined Pork Loin

This succulent recipe tastes great, but because soy sauce is so salty and this marinade contains a lot, I made an adjustment to Ariane's recipe and used low-sodium soy sauce instead of regular soy sauce.

Serves 8 (big portions!) to 12

5-pound pork loin	10 sprigs thyme
2 cups fresh orange juice	¼ cup salt
10 cloves garlic, smashed	½ cup honey
1 cup low-sodium soy sauce	

1. Put the pork loin in a baking dish or plastic resealable bag. Mix the remaining ingredients together in a bowl and pour over the pork loin. Let it sit in the refrigerator overnight.

2. When you are ready to cook, preheat the oven to 500°F. Put the pork and its marinade in a baking dish (if it isn't already) and put it in the oven for 15 minutes. Lower the oven temperature to 325°F and let the pork continue to roast for another 30 to 40 minutes. A meat thermometer inserted into the center of the pork loin should read 160°F when you take it out of the oven. Let it rest for about 20 minutes, then slice and serve.

~~~~~~~~ USE-WHAT-YOU-HAVE VARIATIONS ~~~~~~~~

Use any of these variations, or mix and match them according to your tastes.

VARIATION 1:   Instead of the pork loin, try:
~ Beef tenderloin ~ A large salmon fillet ~ 4 pounds of extra-firm tofu, drained and cut into 16 slices (to serve 8).

VARIATION 2:   Instead of fresh orange juice, try any other citrus juice.

VARIATION 3:   Instead of garlic cloves, try ¼ cup garlic powder or 3 inches fresh ginger, peeled and cut into disks.

VARIATION 4:   Instead of soy sauce, try Worcestershire sauce or low-sodium teriyaki sauce.

VARIATION 5:   Instead of thyme sprigs, try any other fresh herb sprigs, such as rosemary, savory, or marjoram.

VARIATION 6:   Instead of honey, try any other natural liquid sweetener.

~~~~~~

WHAT THE SPRIG?

Sometimes a recipe will call for an herb sprig. A sprig is a piece of the herb, with the stem and leaves attached. They are often used to flavor marinades. Some common examples of herb sprigs are thyme, rosemary, savory, oregano, and marjoram. Often, they don't go into the actual dish, or you fish them out before you serve it. (You can also rub the leaves off the sprigs and use them like you would fresh herbs.) When a recipe calls for a sprig of some herb, you can usually substitute a sprig of a different herb, with the possible exception of mint, which would be too overpowering for most savory dishes.

Creamy Cauliflower Puree

Ariane uses luxurious heavy cream in this recipe, but I've slimmed it down just a little by substituting low-fat milk. Of course, the version that won the *Top Chef* challenge used heavy cream, but this version is still delicious—and significantly skinnier.

Serves 8

*1 head cauliflower, cut into
large pieces
1 Yukon Gold potato, peeled
and cut into large pieces*

*2 cups low-fat milk
Salt and white pepper to taste*

1. Place the cauliflower, potato, milk, salt, and pepper in a pot and cover. Steam slowly for about 20 minutes until the cauliflower and potato are very soft.

2. Remove the cauliflower and potato from the pot and puree them in a food processor until smooth, gradually adding the milk.

~~~~~~~~~ USE-WHAT-YOU-HAVE VARIATIONS ~~~~~~~~~

Use any of these variations, or mix and match them according to your tastes.

VARIATION 1:   Instead of the cauliflower, try 3 extra Yukon Gold potatoes. (Obviously, this will then become a potato puree recipe.)

VARIATION 2:   Instead of the Yukon Gold potato, try any other yellow potato or a red potato.

VARIATION 3:   Instead of low-fat milk, try:
~ Any other plain milk ~ Any plain yogurt.

VARIATION 4:   Instead of white pepper, try black pepper or cayenne pepper.

~~~~~~

Toasted Farro with Garlic Broccoli Rabe and Sun-dried Tomatoes

Farro is an underutilized grain that has a long history and a delicious taste. It is a kind of wheat and it is also sometimes called *emmer*. It is similar but not identical to spelt, with a chewy texture. You're much more likely to see it in Tuscany than in the United States, but lucky you, Ariane has shared her delicious farro recipe with us. You can probably find farro at a natural foods store, or order it online.

Serves 8

½ cup olive oil, divided

2 cups farro

3 cloves garlic, chopped

Salt and pepper to taste

4 cups chicken broth

3 sprigs rosemary

4 cups water

1 teaspoon salt

2 bunches broccoli rabe, stems removed

5 cloves garlic, thinly sliced

1 cup julienned sun-dried tomatoes

2 tablespoons chopped fresh parsley

1. Heat ¼ cup olive oil in a large nonstick skillet over medium heat. Add the farro and let it toast. Add the chopped garlic and season with salt and pepper. Cover with the chicken broth. Add the rosemary sprigs. Lower the heat to medium-low and let cook for about 20 minutes, or until the farro is tender. Remove the rosemary sprigs. Set aside.

2. Boil the water and 1 teaspoon salt in a large saucepan. Add the broccoli rabe and let it cook for about 3 minutes. Remove it from the water with a slotted spoon and put it in a strainer. Shock it by running cold water over it to stop the cooking process. Squeeze out excess water and cut the broccoli rabe into inch-long pieces.

3. Heat ¼ cup olive oil in a sauté pan over medium-high heat and quickly toast the thinly sliced garlic until it turns golden. Add the broccoli rabe, season with more salt and pepper, and add it all to the farro. Finish by sprinkling the sun-dried tomatoes and chopped parsley over the top.

Use any of these variations, or mix and match them according to your tastes.

VARIATION 1: Instead of olive oil, try any other cooking oil.

VARIATION 2: Instead of farro, try:
~ Pearl barley* ~ Spelt* ~ Quinoa.*

VARIATION 3: Instead of chicken broth, try vegetable broth or water.

VARIATION 4: Instead of rosemary sprigs, try any other fresh herb sprigs, such as thyme, savory, or marjoram.

VARIATION 5: Instead of broccoli rabe, try broccolini or broccoli florets.

VARIATION 6: Instead of sun-dried tomatoes, try chopped fresh tomatoes.

VARIATION 7: Instead of parsley, try fresh cilantro.

~~~~~~

Hosea Rosenberg

Hosea won the title of Top Chef on season 5. He's a creative cook, a great guy, and very generous with his recipes. He likes to use local food in his Boulder, Colorado, restaurant, Jax Fish House, so you can always count on him to produce something really fresh and authentic. Of course, his recipes feature seafood—a great Skinnygirl protein source. Find out more about Hosea at www.chefhosea.com.

* Please note that these alternative grains may have different cooking times.

Chilled Avocado Cucumber Soup with Poached Shrimp and Pickled Peppers and Onions

This recipe has luxurious ingredients in three parts, but each part is basically a one-step process, so once you get all your ingredients assembled, you can make this soup in minutes. This recipe calls for a chinoise, which you probably don't have unless you are already a gourmet cook. A chinoise is a cone-shaped sieve with a very fine mesh. If you don't have one, just use a mesh strainer or a few layers of cheesecloth.

Hosea says the garnishes—the shrimp and the pickled peppers and onions— are totally optional, so you can just make the soup and be very happy. If you want to go the whole way, however, the pickled peppers and onions call for a brunoise preparation. You *julienne* them (cut them into matchstick shapes), then cut the matchsticks into cubes so that you get tiny little dice. It takes a while, but it's very easy to do. If you don't have the patience, you can just chop them. The peppers and onions won't look as refined, but they will still taste good.

Serves 6

FOR THE SOUP

3 English cucumbers, peeled
   and chopped

3 avocados, peeled and pitted

1 jalapeño pepper, seeded

¼ cup fresh lemon juice

¼ cup rice vinegar

½ tablespoon sugar

1 tablespoon honey

¼ tablespoon Tabasco sauce

1 cup buttermilk

1 cup water

1½ tablespoons salt

½ cup extra-virgin olive oil

FOR THE SHRIMP

12 medium-size shrimp, shelled
   and cleaned

1 can of your favorite beer

Juice from 2 lemons

1 tablespoon Old Bay Seasoning

2 tablespoons salt

FOR THE PICKLED PEPPERS AND ONIONS

½ red bell pepper, brunoise

½ green bell pepper, brunoise

½ red onion, brunoise

¼ cup sherry vinegar

½ cup red wine vinegar

2 tablespoons sugar

2 bay leaves

Chili-infused oil for garnish

1. Make the soup: Puree all of the soup ingredients except the olive oil in a blender until smooth. Strain through a chinoise. Whisk in the olive oil. Chill and adjust seasoning if necessary.

2. Make the shrimp: Bring all of the shrimp ingredients except the shrimp to a boil. Add the shrimp and cook until just firm and curled, 1 to 2 minutes. Take the shrimp out of the beer mixture and add to an ice bath to chill.

3. Make the pickled peppers and onions: Put the peppers and onion in a plastic container. Bring all of the remaining ingredients except the chili oil to a boil in a saucepan, then pour over the peppers and onion. Cover and let sit at room temperature for 1 hour. Cool. Remove the bay leaves.

4. Put it all together: Pour the soup into cold bowls. Garnish with the poached shrimp and peppers and onion. Drizzle a little chili-infused oil over the top for an extra kick.

~~~~~~~~ USE-WHAT-YOU-HAVE VARIATIONS ~~~~~~~~

Use any of these variations, or mix and match them according to your tastes.

VARIATION 1:   Instead of English cucumbers, try any cucumber, but scrape out all the seeds.

VARIATION 2:   Instead of the fresh jalapeño pepper, try:
~ Pickled jalapeño ~ Chipotle pepper ~ Half of a poblano pepper ~
½ teaspoon red pepper flakes.

VARIATION 3:   Instead of fresh lemon juice, try fresh lime juice.

VARIATION 4:   Instead of rice vinegar, try any other light-colored vinegar.

VARIATION 5:   Instead of sugar, try any other granulated natural sweetener.

VARIATION 6:   Instead of honey, try any other liquid natural sweetener.

VARIATION 7:   Instead of Tabasco sauce, try:
~ Chipotle sauce ~ Any other hot sauce ~ Red pepper flakes.

VARIATION 8:   Instead of buttermilk, try:
~ Greek yogurt ~ Plain soy yogurt ~ Soy milk with 1 teaspoon vinegar
or lemon juice added (let it sit for a few minutes to curdle).

VARIATION 9:   Instead of extra-virgin olive oil, try any other good-quality cold-
pressed oil.

VARIATION 10:   Instead of shrimp, try scallops.

VARIATION 11:   Instead of a can of beer, try 1 cup white wine plus ½ cup water
or 1½ cups water.

VARIATION 12:   Instead of fresh lemon juice, try fresh lime juice.

VARIATION 13:   Instead of Old Bay Seasoning, try any zippy seasoning salt.

VARIATION 14:   Instead of red and green bell peppers, try any other color or
combination of bell peppers.

VARIATION 15:   Instead of red onion, try:
~ Any other onion ~ Leeks ~ Shallots ~ Scallions, white and some green
parts.

VARIATION 16:   Instead of sherry vinegar and red wine vinegar, try:
~ Only sherry or red wine vinegar ~ Any combination of sherry, red
wine, white wine, and champagne vinegar.

VARIATION 17:   Instead of bay leaves, try a sprig of thyme.

~ ~

Dungeness Crab Tian with Mango and Avocado

The term *tian* has come to be known as a layered dish. In Provence, it is like a gratin baked in a tian, which is also the name for the baking dish. People now refer to it more often as a stack of foods. It looks sophisticated and elegant and will impress your guests, but it couldn't be easier.

Even so, a few things in this recipe might give you pause. Hosea will probably want to kick me for saying this, but you can buy really good jumbo lump crabmeat in a can at Costco and probably at other good supermarkets. If I was making this recipe, I would probably use that instead of trying to cook fresh Dungeness crabmeat, even though I'm sure that would be fantastic.

As for the aioli in this recipe, don't be hero. Aioli is a kind of fancy French sauce resembling garlic mayonnaise. Just mince a clove of garlic, mash it up with the side of your chef's knife, and stir it into 2 tablespoons of any good mayonnaise, and call that your aioli.

Serves 4

FOR THE CRAB

8 ounces fresh Dungeness crabmeat

2 tablespoons aioli (see note above)

Zest and juice from 1 lemon

1 teaspoon finely diced chives

½ teaspoon whole-grain mustard

Salt and pepper to taste

FOR THE VANILLA SYRUP (MAKES EXTRA)

1 cup fresh lemon juice

1 cup fresh orange juice

1 cup fresh lime juice

1½ cups sugar

2 vanilla beans, split lengthwise and scraped

FOR THE FINISH

1 ripe mango, diced

1 ripe avocado, diced

1 teaspoon olive oil

1 teaspoon fresh lemon juice

Salt and pepper to taste

Homemade potato chips or crackers for serving

1. Place the crabmeat in a bowl and gently pick through, discarding any shells. In a separate bowl, combine all of the other crab ingredients and slowly fold into the crab, making sure not to break up the crab too much. Taste and adjust the seasoning. Keep cold.

2. Place all of the syrup ingredients in a saucepan and reduce over medium heat until syrupy, about 20 minutes. Strain and cool.

3. Place the mango in the center of a plate. In a bowl, toss the avocado with the olive oil, lemon juice, salt, and pepper and place on top of the mango. Top with the crab. Drizzle a small amount of vanilla syrup around the stack. Serve with homemade potato chips or crackers.

~~~~~~~~~ USE-WHAT-YOU-HAVE VARIATIONS ~~~~~~~~~

Use any of these variations, or mix and match them according to your tastes.

VARIATION 1:   Instead of Dungeness crab, try:
~ Any other kind of cooked crab ~ Small cooked scallops ~ Cooked gulf shrimp ~ Extra-firm tofu, drained and crumbled.

VARIATION 2:   Instead of aioli, try good-quality regular or nondairy mayonnaise.

VARIATION 3:   Instead of fresh lemon juice and zest, try fresh lime juice and zest.

VARIATION 4:   Instead of chives, try scallions, green parts only.

VARIATION 5:   Instead of whole-grain mustard, try any other good mustard.

VARIATION 6:   Instead of lemon, orange, and lime juices, try any other combination of citrus juices.

VARIATION 7:   Instead of sugar, try any other granulated or liquid natural sweetener.

VARIATION 8:   Instead of vanilla beans, try ½ teaspoon real vanilla extract.

VARIATION 9:   Instead of a mango, try:
~ A pear ~ A peach ~ A papaya.

Chile-Citrus Shrimp with Coconut Rice, Gingered Peas, and Red Curry Vinaigrette

This recipe also contains several parts, but they are all quick and easy. Get your ingredients together, do a few quick cooking steps, then put it all together. The only thing I substituted in this recipe is light coconut milk for regular. The light variety has much less fat but the same coconut taste. By the way, chile powder in this recipe refers to pure ground dried red chile peppers. Chili powder, which is a mix of chile and other spices, is different. However, if you don't have or can't find chile powder, chili powder will do.

Serves 4

FOR THE SHRIMP

1½ pounds shrimp, peeled and
    deveined (16 to 20 count)
2 tablespoons chopped fresh
    cilantro
1 tablespoon minced jalapeño
    pepper
2 tablespoons fresh lime
    juice

2 tablespoons fresh lemon

    juice

1 teaspoon chile powder
1 tablespoon soy sauce
1 tablespoon brown sugar
2 teaspoons red pepper
    flakes
1 cup olive oil
Salt and pepper to taste

FOR THE RICE

2 cups water

1 cup jasmine rice, rinsed

1 tablespoon butter

2 tablespoons chopped fresh
  cilantro

½ cup sweetened coconut flakes,
  toasted in a dry skillet until
  golden

½ cup light coconut milk

Salt and pepper to taste

FOR THE PEAS

2 tablespoons canola oil

1 teaspoon minced fresh
  ginger

1 teaspoon minced garlic

2 cups sugar snap peas

2 cups pea shoots

½ teaspoon fresh lime juice

1 tablespoon butter

Salt to taste

FOR THE VINAIGRETTE

3 tablespoons macadamia oil

1 tablespoon rice vinegar

2 teaspoons light coconut milk

2 teaspoons red curry paste

2 teaspoons brown sugar

2 teaspoons orange juice

1 teaspoon lime juice

FOR THE GARNISH

2 tablespoons chopped
  macadamia nuts, toasted
  briefly in a dry skillet until
  golden

2 tablespoons chopped fresh
  cilantro

1. Make the shrimp: Mix all of the shrimp ingredients in a bowl and marinate the shrimp overnight in the refrigerator, then sauté the shrimp in a medium-hot pan just before serving. Season with salt and pepper.

2. Make the rice: Bring the water to a boil. Add the rice and butter and bring to a simmer. Cover until just cooked, about 20 minutes. Transfer the rice to a pan and let cool. When the rice is cool, toss with the cilantro, coconut, and coconut milk. Season with salt and pepper.

3. Make the peas: Heat the canola oil in a nonstick skillet over medium-high heat. Sauté the ginger and garlic for about 1 minute until fragrant. Add the peas and pea shoots and sauté over high heat for about 2 more minutes. Add the lime juice, butter, and salt.

4. Make the vinaigrette: In a bowl combine all of the ingredients and mix well.

5. Put it all together: Warm the rice and place in the center of plates. Arrange the shrimp on top of the rice. Set the sautéed peas to one side. Drizzle the vinaigrette over the shrimp and garnish with the macadamia nuts and cilantro.

~~~~~~~~ USE-WHAT-YOU-HAVE VARIATIONS ~~~~~~~~

Use any of these variations, or mix and match them according to your tastes.

VARIATION 1:   Instead of shrimp, try scallops or extra-firm tofu, drained and cut into scallop shapes.

VARIATION 2:   Instead of cilantro (in any part of the recipe), try any other fresh leafy herb.

VARIATION 3:   Instead of jalapeño, try:
~ Pickled jalapeño ~ Chipotle pepper ~ Half of a poblano pepper.

VARIATION 4:   Instead of lime, lemon, and/or orange juice (in any part of this recipe), try any other citrus juice or combination of citrus juices.

VARIATION 5:   Instead of chile powder, try:
~ Chili powder ~ Ground cumin ~ Paprika.

VARIATION 6:   Instead of soy sauce, try:
~ Tamari ~ Worcestershire sauce ~ Fish sauce ~ Teriyaki sauce.

VARIATION 7:   Instead of brown sugar (in any part of the recipe), try:
~ Raw sugar ~ Agave syrup ~ Real maple syrup.

VARIATION 8:   Instead of red pepper flakes, try cayenne pepper or hot sauce.

VARIATION 9:   Instead of olive oil, try any other cooking oil.

VARIATION 10:   Instead of jasmine rice, try any other rice. (Note different rices may have different cooking time.)

VARIATION 11:   Instead of butter (in any part of the recipe), try nondairy butter or any good-quality cold-pressed oil.

VARIATION 12:   Instead of fresh cilantro, try any other fresh leafy herb.

VARIATION 13:   Instead of sweetened coconut flakes, try unsweetened coconut flakes or fresh grated raw coconut.

VARIATION 14:   Instead of coconut milk (in the rice and vinaigrette), try any other plain milk.

VARIATION 15:   Instead of minced garlic and ginger, try ¼ teaspoon each garlic powder and ground ginger or leaving either one out (but at least try to use one of them, for the great flavor).

VARIATION 16:   Instead of canola oil, try any other cooking oil.

VARIATION 17:   Instead of sugar snap peas, try any other fresh seasonal peas.

VARIATION 18:   Instead of pea shoots, try snow peas, cut in bite-size pieces.

VARIATION 19:   Instead of macadamia oil, try any other nut oil or extra-virgin olive oil.

VARIATION 20:   Instead of rice vinegar, try:
    ~ Champagne vinegar ~ White wine vinegar ~ Dry white wine.

VARIATION 21:   Instead of red curry paste, try:
    ~ Any other curry paste ~ Red chili paste ~ Asian hot sauce (like sriracha).

VARIATION 22:   Instead of macadamia nuts, try any other nut.

Epilogue

As this book comes to a close, I want to thank you with all of my heart for taking this journey with me. Those of you who read my books and watch my shows help to hold me up and keep me focused and grateful. In return, I want to continue to support you in your efforts to feel strong, empowered, and naturally thin.

In that spirit, remember that cooking, just like eating, can become *yours*, not anyone else's, and that a recipe is a thing in flux, not a thing in stone.

Now go out and live your life. Eat well and make every bite worthwhile. Move your body, enjoy your life, and don't waste another minute kicking yourself for making mistakes. When you make a mistake, with a food choice or in the kitchen, it's okay. Do you know why? Because you already did it, so it has to be okay. Notice what happened and move on to the next thing.

Your next investment, your next meal, your next cooking attempt will be a good one, and that's how you'll know you are a true Skinnygirl.

Acknowledgments

Thank you to all of my fans and readers who had the faith in me to purchase *Naturally Thin,* to trust it, and to allow it to change you forever. *The Skinnygirl Dish* was written to teach you how to see your kitchen and cooking in a whole new light.

Thank you to Zach Schisgal and Marcia Burch at Touchstone Fireside for helping me in the entire publishing journey.

Lori Levine, you have been tireless and passionate about my career. And I cannot thank you enough.

Molly Hayden and Julie Plake, you have been dedicated, driven, and such an incredible team to help me bring this book to life. Thanks for knowing how crazy I am and loving me that much more.

Eve Adamson, my cowriter, you are the most patient, calm, and efficient writer who completely "gets" it, me, and anything I want to express. I always write endlessly and give you a mess, and you happily and diligently structure it. You are so talented, and you know so much about everything that is important to me. You are my Bernie Taupin, and this will be a life-long journey, so stay healthy!

Jason Hoppy, thank you for loving me despite how intense and type A I am. Thank you for being the most decent, kind, loving, and supportive man a woman could ever hope to find. You make me stronger and happier, you give me hope, and you show me that all dreams can come true and you can have it all.

Cookie aka Dabooboo, you are my best friend, furry or otherwise. You are the sweetest, cutest, most complicated canine God could ever have created. You have loved me, snuggled me, and supported me throughout everything I do.

Xoxo

Index

Spanish spiced rubbed chicken with
    mustard-green onion sauce,
    249–52
spice rub, Spanish, 251
spices, 31, 65, 66
    how and when to grind, 80–81
    how to use, 79–80
Spike seasoning, 77
spinach:
    and artichoke dip, guilt-free, 239–41
    and artichoke dip, guilt-free (with
      substitutes), 50–52
    with white bean soup, 116–17
spreads, 28, 38, 234
    for burgers, 105
    for sandwiches, 104, 114
springform pans, 182
Starbucks, 95
stevia, 56
stirring, 77
stocks, purchased, 35, 36
Strawberry Daiquiris, Skinnygirl,
    227
stuffing, Skinnygirl rice, 214–15
substitutes, food:
    baking, 56–57
    cocktails, 57
    dairy products, 55
    grains, nuts, and seeds, 54
    guilt-free artichoke and spinach dip,
      50–52
    oil, vinegars, and citrus, 55–56
    tofu as, 24, 43–44
    vegetable and fruit, 53–54
succotash, summer, with seared diver
    scallops and orange gastrique,
    262–64
sugar, white vs. raw, 179
Sutter, Ryan, 90
Sutter, Trista, 90
sweeteners, 29, 56, 172, 179
sweet potato(es):
    mashed, 132–34, 203
    soufflé, 216

tacos, healthy, 137–38
tapenade, 37, 104
Today show, 174, 268
tofu, 24, 43–44
    basic preparation of, 75–76
tomato(es), 26
    roasted, and arugula, seared
      watermelon salad with, 265–66
    soup, sweet, 119–20
    sun-dried, mozzarella, and arugula
      panini, 109–11
    sun-dried, toasted farro with garlic
      broccoli rabe and, 271–72
    -watermelon vinaigrette, 267
    whole-grain bruschetta with fresh
      basil and, 160–61
tomato sauce, canned, 37
Top Chef series, 248, 257, 268
top chefs' recipes, 248–81
    chile-citrus shrimp with coconut rice,
      gingered peas, and red curry
      vinaigrette, 278–81
    chilled avocado cucumber soup with
      poached shrimp and pickled
      peppers and onions, 273–75
    creamy cauliflower puree, 270
    Dungeness crab tian with mango and
      avocado, 276–77
    grilled basil-rubbed pork chops with
      grilled nectarine–blue cheese salad
      and toasted pignoli nuts, 253–55
    orange juice brined pork loin, 268–69
    seared diver scallops, summer
      succotash, and orange gastrique,
      262–64
    seared watermelon salad with roasted
      tomatoes and arugula, 265–66
    slow-roasted salmon with herb
      vinaigrette, 255–57
    Spanish spiced rubbed chicken with
      mustard-green onion sauce,
      249–52
    steamed bass with root vegetable salad
      and ponzu sauce, 258–62

"Bethenny Frankel's book promises—and delivers—the ultimate dream of every overweight American: that you can be 'naturally thin' without starvation dieting, exercising like a maniac, taking drugs, or feeling hungry all the time."

—Ellen Kunes, editor in chief, *Health* magazine

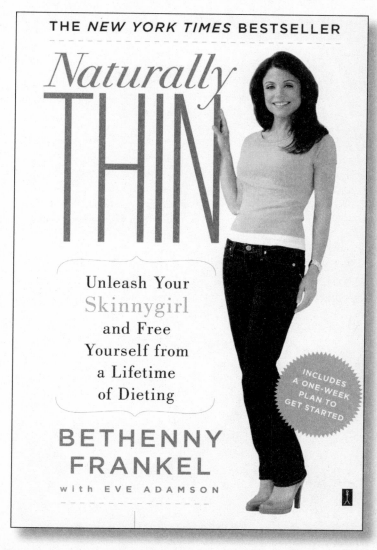

Available wherever books are sold or at www.simonandschuster.com

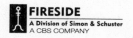